THE TWENTY-FOUR HOUR MIND

The Twenty-four Hour Mind

The Role of Sleep and Dreaming in

Our Emotional Lives

Rosalind D. Cartwright

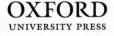

OXFORD
UNIVERSITY PRESS

2010

OXFORD
UNIVERSITY PRESS

Oxford University Press, Inc., publishes works that further
Oxford University's objective of excellence
in research, scholarship, and education.

Oxford   New York
Auckland   Cape Town   Dar es Salaam   Hong Kong   Karachi
Kuala Lumpur   Madrid   Melbourne   Mexico City   Nairobi
New Delhi   Shanghai   Taipei   Toronto

With offices in
Argentina   Austria   Brazil   Chile   Czech Republic   France   Greece
Guatemala   Hungary   Italy   Japan   Poland   Portugal   Singapore
South Korea   Switzerland   Thailand   Turkey   Ukraine   Vietnam

Copyright © 2010, by Oxford University Press, Inc.

Published by Oxford University Press, Inc.
198 Madison Avenue, New York, New York 10016
www.oup.com
Oxford is a registered trademark of Oxford University Press

Library of Congress Cataloging-in-Publication Data
Cartwright, Rosalind Dymond.
The twenty-four hour mind : the role of sleep and dreaming in our emotional lives/
Rosalind D. Cartwright.
p. cm.
Includes bibliographical references.
ISBN 978-0-19-538683-7 (hardback : acid-free paper) 1. Sleep—Research.
2. Sleep disorders. I. Title.
RA786.C37 2010
616.2'090072—dc22   2009045764

3 5 7 9 8 6 4 2

Printed in the United States of America
on acid-free paper

*To all those who have brought the
light of science to illuminate
the dark of night*

Acknowledgments

No book is the product of a single author; this one owes its existence to many others. Dreams are free but their scientific study is not. It takes equipment, space and time, technicians to monitor the sleepers, and research assistants to do all the chores that come afterward. Frank Diaz and Graciella Padilla were enormously helpful techs and Paul Newell, Pat Mercer, Michael Bears, Erin Baer, Ellen Wood, and Steve Lloyd were all important contributors as we worked together. Funding for this work from the National Institute of Mental Health made possible the longitudinal studies of depression. Institutional support came from the dean and now president of Rush University, Larry Goodman. My thinking about the function of REM sleep and dreaming was deeply influenced by Allan Rectschaffen, Chris Gillin, Milton Kramer, Gerry Vogel, Ray Greenberg, and Ernie Hartmann. Others to thank are those whose work on sleepwalking, under Jacques Montplaisir, have been invaluable, as was the collaboration of Christian Guilleminault who loaned his expertise in spectral analysis scoring for two of the cases cited in this book. There are two other central players to thank: Scott Falater, serving a life sentence for the fatal attack on his wife, and Sarah Harrington, my editor. By allowing his case and subsequent dreams to be included, Scott trusts the reader to consider the validity of his sleepwalking defense. And, Sarah, my editor, while trusting my vision of the continuously working mind, has prodded me to clarify my thinking.

Her skillful editing has smoothed the sentence structure, and shortened and sharpened the text, helping this to become a more coherent whole. It is now a road map through the normal progression of the mind's work from day into night as this is illuminated by the effects of specific disruptions from several sleep disorders.

Contents

Introduction

The idea that sleep is good for us, beneficial to both mind and body, lies behind the classic advice from the busy physician: "Take two aspirins and call me in the morning." But the meaning of this message is somewhat ambiguous. Will a night's sleep plus the aspirin be of help no matter what ails us, or does the doctor himself need a night's sleep before he is able to dispense more specific advice? In either case, the presumption is that there is some healing power in sleep for the patient or better insight into the diagnosis for the doctor, and that the overnight delay allows time for one or both of these natural processes to take place. Sometimes this happens, but unfortunately sometimes it does not. Sometimes it is sleep itself that is the problem.

Our understanding of just what sleep does for us has advanced considerably over the last few decades. The modern era of sleep research began in a small way in the 1950s, when a University of Chicago physiologist named Nathaniel Kleitman pioneered a method for investigating what happens in both the brain and body while we sleep. He started by paying healthy male medical students ten dollars a night to sleep under observation in his laboratory while wearing electrodes that would record their brain waves and eye movements. This turned out to be a real bargain, because what Kleitman and his assistants found was the start of a whole new field of research that opened the black box of sleep to the light of science.

The first finding that came from these all-night vigils was that, contrary to previous belief, sleep is not a time-out of uniform unconsciousness in which nothing much goes on until we wake up. Sleep is not a state of coma, but rather a period of regular cyclic changes between two distinctive organizations of brain and body activity. These two types of sleep are as different from each other as sleep is from waking. Quiet sleep comes first, then the body's major physiological systems tune down for a period of rest that looks for all the world as if the body is about to enter a state of hibernation. Heart rate slows down, as does respiration, and body temperature begins to fall. In the brain, electrical activity also slows, and brain waves change from the rapid rate of waking to high-amplitude slow waves as sleep deepens. After about an hour and a half, this whole picture changes and active sleep takes over. The body's systems shift back into high gear, except for the major muscles that control movement; these relax abruptly while the eyes begin to move rapidly behind closed lids. It is then, while the body is limp and unable to move, that the mind produces the hallucinations that we call dreams.

Dreaming captured the attention of clinicians and researchers when the fruits of Kleitman's laboratory work were first published in two landmark papers in 1953 and 1955. Psychotherapists were excited by the prospect that Kleitman's technology would yield much more information than patients could remember of their dreams on their own. They hoped this would help them to get closer to the roots of the hidden anxieties and motivations that undermined their patients' own best interests. Could this new sleep research speed the long, tough work of uncovering the origin of psychological symptoms hidden in the unconscious?

Stimulated by Kleitman's discoveries, scientists from many disciplines turned to sleep as a new area to explore. They took two different routes. Neuroscientists took a "bottom-up" approach, recording activity deep in the brain cells of rats and cats in order to discover where active sleep (termed REM, for rapid eye movement) originated, to map where and how it turned on in the brain stem, and to follow its path up to where it stimulates the eyes to dart about rapidly.

Psychologists and psychiatrists, on the other hand, started at the "top," investigating the dream experience of human volunteers by waking them out of each of the three, four, or five REM periods, depending on how long they slept, to hear their reports of what they had been experiencing. They pondered on why we spend so much sleep time engaged in this bizarre hallucinatory behavior. The first dream experiments focused on this question, trying to tease out the purpose of dreaming by testing what happened when REM sleep was selectively suppressed. Did humans become psychotic if they were not allowed to hallucinate safely in sleep? Did dreams keep us sane?

Both the neuroscientists' bottom-up and psychologists' top-down research approaches to understanding sleep paid off with a tremendous body of new information. But neither route settled our most basic questions about the meaning and functions of dreams—or if, in fact, they had either. A lively debate began between these two camps that continues to this day: Are dreams an important source of information about the mind, or are they just a random by-product of periodically heightened brain activity, with no specific meaning at all? Many theories were proposed; one suggested that the rapid eye movements only occur because the brain is exercising the eyes in order to keep binocular vision ready to go to work, in case there comes a need to focus quickly in an emergency.

The debate about whether REM has any psychological function has lost some of its steam as research over the last 10 years showed that quiet sleep, called non-REM (NREM) and active REM sleep both appear to be integral to—and to cooperate in—the consolidation and conversion of new learning into long-term memory. Each type of sleep may have other functions, just as our waking minds perform in many ways, but in this crucial aspect of the mind's work in storing new experience, the two sleep types are interdependent, as we shall see.

A second debate, still active, is whether dreaming is dependent on REM sleep or if it is an independent type of mental life ongoing throughout all sleep—perhaps dreams are simply more easily recalled when the brain state is highly active (during REM) and is cut off for a time from the outside world. Some of this debate rests on the difference in various definitions of a dream. Those who broadly define dreams as any mental activity sleepers recall when they are awakened believe "dreaming" goes on in all but the deepest stages of sleep. Others stick to the definition of a dream as a sensory experience, mostly visual but with other senses involved, connected by a narrative structure that we believe to be real at the time, no matter how bizarre. Using this definition, dreams are largely confined to REM sleep. I favor this narrower definition of a dream, but acknowledge that such dreams can be harvested from NREM sleep in some people and under some circumstances. Light sleepers are one such group, as are those who are REM deprived, and almost anyone when in a highly anxious state. Dreams can not be a random by-product of REM sleep if they can also occur in NREM sleep. The unique eye movements and loss of muscle tone of REM sleep together provide the ideal signal for identifying when dreams can be most systematically sampled for further study. What is sampled from NREM awakenings is more often single images or random thoughts.

Disagreement in the scientific community about the importance of study-ing dreams continues to be lively, and there is no shortage of interesting research questions and volunteers willing to participate in studies and to aid us in our continuing search to understand what we dream about and why. For instance, many brain-injured patients will notice specific changes to their dreams depending on the part of the brain that has been damaged. Some experience a lack of color in the dream images, or they find that, following the injury, their dreams no longer feature any people. Or, they may cease to have any dreams at all. Knowing the regions of the brain that are affected by a given injury, changes in dream characteristics help scientists map how and where dreams are constructed.

Some 20 years after the initial flood of studies on the sleep of rats, cats, and healthy young men, the same monitoring techniques Kleitman pioneered began to be applied to the study of troubled sleepers, and a whole new branch of medicine was born. Sleep medicine is devoted to the understanding and treatment of a host of newly identified disorders that came to light when researchers began studying the sleep of patients complaining of sleep troubles. The common complaint of insomnia ("I just can't seem to get enough sleep any more") turned out to be as nonspecific as "I'm running a fever." So did the opposite complaint—"I fall asleep all the time, at work, while driving, over TV." Too little sleep might be due to anything from a bad habit, to an addiction to late night surfing of the web, to major depression. Too much daytime sleepiness also has various causes: It might be a symptom of narcolepsy or sleep apnea, a hangover from some new medicine, or simply the result of not getting enough nighttime sleep.

As soon as the host of new sleep disorders was identified and confirmed in many labs, it became clear that the field needed to develop a manual that would define and systematize their diagnosis. Sleep disorders research became a hot topic because of the potential for clinical application of basic research, and because sleep problems were so under-attended and debilitating. Studies reported that short hours of sleep make us not only less attentive, slower to learn, more likely to make mistakes, and more accident prone (which most of us can attest to), but also cause us to have shorter tempers, to be more open to infections, to put on weight, and to die sooner than we should.

The last few years have also seen a tremendous increase in media coverage of sleep research findings and in advertising dollars devoted to promoting products promising a good night's sleep—so much that the twenty-first century might well be called "The Century of Sleep." With sleep thrust into the spotlight, mattress companies began innovating to improve sleep by individualizing their products to deliver a unique cocoon of comfort. Other ads informed us that if the snoring of our bed partner disturbed our sleep, we could have the offender fitted with a dental appliance that would quiet the noise, so that we could again enjoy sharing the bed, along with its new individualized comfort mattress.

By far, the industry that has most enthusiastically embraced the importance of sleep is the drug business. Pharmaceutical companies responded to the news of how many suffer with insomnia by offering newer, safer, non-narcotic sleep aids, assuring consumers that they would wake up smiling, ready to face whatever comes their way the next day. The number of prescriptions dispensed for sleep medicines has soared in the past dozen years, undeterred by side effects that have surfaced. Recently, a rash of news stories told of some sleep aid users getting up from bed shortly after falling asleep and then acting in a most unusual fashion. Not only were these sleepwalkers unaware that what they were doing at the time was not rational, they had no memory of what they had done the next morning. Some headed for the kitchen, cooking and sometimes eating bizarre combinations of foods—packages of unbaked cookie mix, for example. Or they headed out to shop, driving to the store still in their pajamas. Others climbed to dangerous heights and were spotted curled up asleep on top of bridges or construction cranes. Many of these were initially considered amusing isolated incidents, but there were others of a more serious nature. Attempts at sexual contact with a sleeping child resulted in the arrest of more than one apparently upright citizen.

After enough reports of sleep-aid–related violence, like a vicious beating or a stabbing of a loved one, the U.S. Food and Drug Administration (FDA) acted. The agency required that two famous sleeping pill makers add to their labels and advertising copy a warning that sleepwalking, sleep eating, sleep driving, and sleep sex may occur as side effects. This is a case where the treatment of a sleep disorder turned out to be potentially more dangerous than the disorder it was designed to correct. It underlined the importance of a proper diagnosis that must precede treatment, and that, in order to understand and treat sleep problems, we must first better understand what is happening in the sleeping body and brain.

Until recently, insomnia had been slow to get research attention in part because the prescription pad was too handy a solution—on the surface, insomnia responds quickly to pharmaceutical treatment, and partly also because insomnia is so common that it was treated like the common cold—"wait a while and it will go away." Now that insomnia has been recognized as a major risk factor for a number of health problems, there has been an appropriate shift away from band-aiding it with a pill and toward serious investigation. This research has uncovered a strong association between sleep of poor quality and reduced quantity and some of our most major medical problems, including obesity, diabetes, hypertension, heart attacks, and stroke. Poor sleep quality and short duration have also been linked to the development of mental health problems, specifically major depression and anxiety disorders.

Although there are countless fascinating paths one might choose to go down in a book about sleep, this one is devoted to connecting what we know of the mind awake with what we have learned from research into the mind asleep. More specifically, what can dreams and behavior during sleep tell us about our waking selves, and what clues about our physical and mental health can be discovered by studying our sleep? Sleep disorders and mood disorders have been a focus of my own research and treatment work for many years. My more recent involvement with serious sleepwalking cases has introduced me to another role of sleep scientists—testifying as a sleep expert in courtroom cases of sleepwalking aggression or sexual behaviors. If a sleepwalker is not in a conscious state of mind during an aggressive act, is he or she legally responsible for the consequences of their behavior? How sure can we be of the diagnosis? Can dreams play a role in illuminating the hidden motives behind the behavior of sleepwalkers?

I will lay out a new psychological model of the twenty-four hour mind; that is, how the predominantly conscious (waking) and unconscious (sleeping) forms of mental behavior interact throughout the brain's regular, but differently organized, states of waking, sleeping, and dreaming. This is based on my own work, as well as that of many others who have contributed to a "horizontal" approach to understanding the human mind. We know now that the brain does not simply turn off when we switch off the bedside lamp; rather, it continues to be active. However, the brain's night-shift involves a different set of chores than those of the daytime hours. As we move through 16 hours of wake time, mostly we are paying attention to and interacting with the outside world. When we shut down that input for 8 hours of sleep, the brain begins selecting from the waking hours those new experiences to be kept active, so that they may be filed into memory. My research has led me to add to this model the idea that while dreaming we are also down-regulating any disruptive emotions attached to those new experiences and modifying the software program of the self on the basis of this new information (it is this "self system" which guides much of our waking behavior). This wake–sleep collaboration is how our behavior remains flexible, how we are able to retain new learning and safely negotiate the bumps of unanticipated misfortunes. This process works well only if sleep is intact, regular, and long enough to complete its nightly tasks. When sleep is not optimal in these ways, difficulties both large and small may occur. I will illustrate these interactions with case examples throughout the book.

Come along. I promise this will be an interesting ride.

THE TWENTY-FOUR HOUR MIND

In the Beginning: The Early Days of Sleep Research

I have an exposition of sleep come upon me.

—William Shakespeare, *A Midsummer Night's Dream*

Psychology, the science of human behavior, is constantly reinventing itself. In the early 1930s, as psychology was breaking away from its parents, philosophy and physiology, and defining itself as a separate discipline, it took as its mission the scientific study of three areas: cognition, conation, and affection. That is the way I learned the terms as an undergrad in 1941, and as I later discovered, they translated into more modern usage as thinking, motivation, and emotion. At the time, these were treated as separate fields for investigation. It took the research referred to as the "new look in perception" in the 1950s for the interactions of these processes to begin to be recognized; that even what and how we see is guided by what we want at the time (motivation), and how we evaluate (feel about) it. Psychology, then, had its hands full focusing on understanding those conscious mental processes that make us uniquely intelligent, able to think before we act, to choose what is on our mind, to learn from experience, and to remember what we learn.

In the past, the most popular topics of inquiry for students of psychology were questions about failure, or dysfunction—why we sometimes fail to think clearly, are slow to learn, act impulsively, and in general mess up. Courses in abnormal psychology were (and still are) taught in many academic programs; but to distinguish psychology from psychiatry, and particularly from psycho-analysis (which was flourishing in the 1950s) academic psychologists around midcentury studiously avoided studying the role of unconscious thinking, motivation, or emotion, as explanations for strange behavior. The term "unconscious" itself was treated as a historic relic adopted before scientific methods were developed for the empirical investigation of human behavior. After all, how can we study something we cannot see, feel, or measure?

I remember in my first classes at the university hearing the emphasis on that word, "empirical," and not understanding its meaning. I quickly learned all that it entailed: that the questions asked by psychologists should be only those that could be answered by the methods of science, yielding objective proof. That principle ruled out the unconscious as an explanatory term but left a lot of interesting questions about why we do not always use our cognitive abilities to our best advantage.

Take the classic Jack Benny joke, for example. When asked by a hold-up man, "Your money or your life?" Benny takes a very long pause, then when prodded responds "I'm thinking." What is it about this picture that makes us laugh? We realize that something beyond thinking is at issue under this circumstance—that something more than cognition—emotion—is involved in making his choice, and Benny's audience appreciates this. "Thinking" should lead to a conclusion, a choice, but Benny is stopped cold, unable to decide between two alternatives, as both are highly valued. We do not always use our highest mental abilities, but instead run on what we could call "automatic pilot"; once learned, many of our daily cognitive behaviors are directed by habit, those already-formed points of view, attitudes, and schemas that in part make us who we are. The formation of these habits frees us to use our highest mental processes for those special instances when a prepared response will not do, when circumstances change and attention must be paid, choices made or a new response developed. The result is that much of our baseline thoughts and behavior operate unconsciously.

Jack Benny's dilemma is a case in which he has no prepared easy answer, and his rational decision-making process has been hijacked by emotion. When emotion gets the better of us—when we fall in love or into despair, act out of anger or freeze in fear, then our emotions may make us act irrationally for a time. We later explain this to ourselves and others by saying, "I just wasn't thinking." These are the exceptions to our usual access to high-order thinking when needed, and a clue about the importance of the unconscious. Typically, we switch back and forth between being fully conscious—alert and focused—and being *potentially* conscious while on auto-pilot, like driving a familiar route until we spot a police car tailing behind us. That gets our focused attention, and also a sinking feeling of anxiety.

How does this talk about the unconscious relate to sleep and dreams? When emotions evoked by a waking experience are strong, or more often were under-attended at the time they occurred, they may not be fully resolved by nighttime. In other words, it may take us a while to come to terms with strong or neglected emotions. If, during the day, some event challenges a basic, habitual way in which we think about ourselves (such as the comment from a friend, "Aren't you putting on weight?") it may be a threat to our self-concepts. It will probably be brushed off at the time, but that question, along with its emotional baggage, will be carried forward in our minds into sleep. Nowadays, researchers do not stop our investigations at the border of sleep but continue to trace mental activity from the beginning of sleep on into dreaming. All day, the conscious mind goes about its work planning, remembering, and choosing, or just keeping the shop running as usual. On balance, we humans are more action oriented by day. We stay busy doing, but in the inaction of sleep we turn inward to review and evaluate the implications of our day, and the input of those new perceptions, learnings, and—most important—emotions about what we have experienced.

What we experience as a dream is the result of our brain's effort to match recent, emotion-evoking events to other similar experiences already stored in long-term memory. One purpose of this sleep-related matching process, this putting of similar memory experiences together, is to defuse the impact of those feelings that might otherwise linger and disrupt our moods and behaviors the next day. The various ways in which this extraordinary mind of ours works— the top-level rational thinking and executive deciding functions, the middle management of routine habits of thought, and the emotional relating and updating of the organized schemas of our self-concept—are not isolated from each other. They interact. The emotional aspect, which is often not consciously recognized, drives the not-conscious mental activity of sleep. This is what is new—and the nature of the unconscious needs to be studied if we are to understand human behavior fully.

Recently psychological experiments into decision making have rediscovered that unconscious activity is ongoing during waking, and that this can be studied with well-controlled research designs. Several teams of psychologists in Europe and now in the United States have begun to explore what unconscious cognition does, and especially what it does in some circumstances even better than high-level conscious thought. For example, when we stop trying hard to solve a puzzle or remember a name, the right answer often pops up later, while we are engaged in doing something else. This new interest in unconscious thinking as it affects waking choices and the scientific study of the mind in sleep are ready to be joined to give us a fuller picture of the human psyche.

Let me begin with some observations on my own intertwining of conscious and unconscious thought, which helped bring me to this point of view. Some nights when sleep does not arrive promptly, I find my mind takes off on its own and without my direction, reviews "what's new" and evaluates "how I'm doing." What came into my mind on one such recent night was a nickname I acquired many years ago: "The Queen of Dreams." I laughed to myself, thinking, "You can't be the Queen of Dreams if you don't get to sleep." Suddenly, another name popped up, "The House of Sacred Sleep." That was a name we children gave to our family home as a joke, shared at my mother's expense. I had not thought of it in years. Then I saw the link between these two "random" thoughts: my self-criticism for not living up to the title bestowed on me following a talk on the function of dreams; and the positive value I placed on good sleep inspired by my mother's conviction of its healing power. That emotional connection acted as a key, unlocking a closet full of memories. Now it was clear to me why I had focused my research on what happens in the mind at night. After many years as a sleep scientist, I am convinced that the time has come to put together what I and many others have learned of the sleeping mind with what psychologists know of waking cognitive and emotional behaviors.

More than a hundred years ago, Sigmund Freud made an attempt to spell out an integrative model of the psyche in his "Project for a Scientific Psychology"; this was before he wrote the book for which he is best known, *The Interpretation of Dreams*. Freud gave up his "Project," realizing that, as a neurologist, he could not produce scientific proof of his theory, handicapped as he was before the turn of the century by the lack of tools for investigating the neuronal connections he was proposing as the basis of the unconscious. He took another route, listening to what his patients could recall of their dreams, convinced that these were an expression of the unconscious. From this, he built his three-layered dynamic model of the mind. Freud was not naïve enough to believe these layers of the mind had actual brain locations, but used them as an easy way to convey his ideas. The bottom layer was the largest and contained the oldest parts of the human psyche. Here are the inherited primitive motives responsible for our survival; the drives of hunger to maintain the body, aggression to fend off enemies, exploration of new territory, and sex to ensure a next generation. All of these Freud believed were only partially tamed in their expression by our learning the "polite," socially acceptable ways to get these motives satisfied. These he believed remain active in their original form throughout life. Although unconscious, they can be observed in their disguised expression in dreams. Above the bottom archaic material, in the second layer lies the preconscious mind, which holds memories that can be brought into focus by turning our attention on them. This preconscious is in touch with both the unconscious and conscious. The third layer of this model and the smallest area, the conscious mind, is what we are aware of seeing, feeling, remembering, and wanting in the present.

Now that we have the brain monitoring equipment Freud lacked, we can begin to tackle the task of putting together what we have learned of the waking mind with what we know of the mental activity of our "off hours" of sleep. With this, we can revisit one of sleep research's long-lasting debates: Where do we go when we go to sleep? With rare exceptions, older academicians held that in sleep we sink into a nonconscious oblivion that we can safely disregard as unimportant to understanding our waking lives. To me, it is clear that in sleep there is continuing mental functioning that operates behind our backs and out of our control, but which has a powerful interaction with our waking life. Much of what Freud intuited about the meaning and function of dreams can now be formally tested, but over and above that are the many new findings from both research into the waking mind and sleep research, which can be used to develop a new working model of the twenty-four hour mind.

I believe that the night mind has its own special tasks that help keep us on an even emotional keel (at least when it is working properly). Like all of our natural processes—digestion, for example, which can become indigestion—sleep can malfunction. Sleepwalking, for example, is important to our new model because it is a condition in which the mind is functioning in a combined sleep/wake state, where unconscious motives are driving physical behavior, without consciousness at the time and without memory of the event after waking consciousness returns. From this we can observe in overt behavior what the mind/brain has going on in sleep, despite the lack of oversight from our higher processes due to the continuing unconsciousness of sleep.

Major depression is another instructive disorder characterized by, among other symptoms, disturbed sleep and dreaming. The rapid eye movement (REM) sleep in those who are suffering a major depression is misplaced in its timing in the sleep–wake cycle. The first opportunity to dream occurs too soon, and with an abnormal frequency of eye movements in many of those suffering with this disorder. This too-early and too-active REM, first noted by David Kupfer of the University of Pittsburgh, displaces some of the restful non-REM (NREM) sleep that usually precedes it. In severe depression, dreaming is often devoid of any coherent narrative thread, but in milder depression dreams express emotions that have become flat, and a dreamed self that is passive and lacking responsiveness. When the emotional component of the dream story shifts within the night from being negative in the first hours to positive in the late hours—from anxiety or unhappiness to pleasure or joyful expectation—and the images in the dream story include the waking emotional concerns melded with related older memories, making a patchwork of old and new images difficult to understand, a healthy process is actually under way. Sleepwalking and major depression give us unique windows into the role of sleep in our emotional health. They also furnish us with a better understanding of the early warning signs of mental health troubles that often show up first as disordered sleep.

Before I became a sleep scientist, I grew up believing that sleep is a built-in physician and dreams an internal psychotherapist; that good sleep rests and restores our weary bodies and that good dreams temper our emotional responses to new experiences. Now hard evidence supports those assumptions, that adequate sleep is essential to physical health, and that dreaming is important to mental health. When we short-cut our sleep, as many of us are wont to do these days, neither sleep nor dreams can perform their functions fully.

How Sleep Researcher Became the "Leading Lady" Part of My Self-concept

When it came time to choose a career, I could find no academic program that would allow me to explore the world of sleep; none of the college catalogs I sent for listed any relevant courses. Freud was by then considered "old hat." Nonetheless I found psychology to be a natural fit, and after obtaining a doctorate I settled into a position on a research team at the University of Chicago with Carl Rogers, who was testing the efficacy of his new client-centered psychotherapy. This technique trained therapists to stay in the moment with their clients, and not to probe into where dysfunctional attitudes and behaviors came from. This was a strong departure from the psychoanalytic method, which actively sought the unconscious childhood roots of dysfunctional symptoms like depression and anxiety. Rogers taught therapists to "follow the feelings," in order to help clients to experience and articulate their emotions. While the psychoanalysts targeted unconscious impulses from the past by analyzing patients' dreams, Rogers's target was those almost-conscious emotions that lay "at the edge of awareness."

As luck would have it, my secretary Pat was dating a medical student who worked nights as a laboratory assistant for Nathaniel Kleitman, the acknowledged father of sleep research. One day, she came in breathlessly excited, dropped down in the chair beside my desk, and said, "Did you know that peoples' eyes move when they are dreaming?" The medical student, whom she later married, was Bill Dement, and he along with Eugene Aserinsky and Dr. Kleitman published the first research papers showing that dreaming was detectable in a distinctive pattern of active brain waves, looking almost like waking, and in the rapid eye movements in sleeping volunteers. They called their discovery REM sleep, and it opened the magical world of dreams to serious scientific exploration.

I confess I did not appreciate at the time the opportunity Pat offered me with that breaking news. I was too committed then to the job I already had, which did not include studying dreaming as a link to the unconscious. In fact, it was another ten years, after Rogers and I published a book reporting the results of our work, before I was ready to tackle a new area of research. It was then that I remembered that the field of dreams was turf I could now plow.

I was at that time Director of Psychology at the University of Illinois Medical College. I created my first sleep lab there by commandeering part of a men's bathroom in an unused psychiatric unit turned office space. There were two separate tub rooms adjacent to the urinals. I replaced the bathtubs with beds and installed an intercom system and the electrical shielding and wiring needed to carry signals from the monitors worn by the sleepers to a control room next door. In this control room two modified electroencephalograph (EEG) machines were installed to record the brain waves, eye movements, and heart rates of the sleepers—and just enough room for a newly minted PhD colleague and me to sit up on stools all night watching the pens trace on rolls of paper the brain waves of our two sleeping volunteers. Each night, we waited for the distinctive signs of REM to appear before calling on the intercom to ask the sleepers to tell us what was happening in their minds. We never asked about "dreams," as that would bias the response.

From study to study, I worked at getting funding where I could, writing up research results, traveling to meetings to learn about the work of others, and sharing what I was finding. I joined the small band of sleep-watchers that made up a network of friends that reached around the world. I felt like a member of a nocturnal secret society.

In the early days, or rather nights, I did many different kinds of studies. One experiment investigated whether the hallucinations volunteers experienced after being injected with an experimental drug (it was the '60s) resembled the images they produced naturally in their dreams. I wanted to know if we could use a drug to induce dreaming while the volunteers were awake and better able to tell me what was happening at the time.

One of the inherent flaws in sleep and dream research is that, by awakening the sleeping volunteer to ask for a report, we forever alter the course of that night's natural mental activity. By changing their state to waking, sleepers become conscious of their reports, which might well influence what they tell us at the next REM opportunity. Also, waking the sleeper from each REM period means we sacrifice hearing the end of the story. We have no choice but to interrupt the sleepers while they are still experiencing REM sleep, as the memory of dreams fades quickly once that sleep episode is over and sleepers descend into another NREM sleep cycle (Fig. 1.1). The next time REM sleep appears, some 90 minutes later, the dreamers' reports may have a similar theme, but it will be embedded in a different story using different images.

I had another purpose for undertaking that experimental drug study. Bill Dement had published a few years earlier, in 1960, a block-buster article showing that if REM sleep is suppressed for a few nights by waking the sleeper each time this stage of sleep is about to begin, the sleeping brain tries more and more urgently to initiate REM. Not just the typical three or four times a night must the sleeper be wakened; pressure for REM builds faster in some people than in others, but it might take as many as thirty awakenings a night to prevent REM from happening. The big news from this study was that once these volunteers were released to sleep without any interruption, they had a major "REM bash." For the next few nights, the proportion of their REM sleep was higher than usual. This was interpreted at the time as showing that people need to dream, with a steady average of 20%–25% of sleep spent in REM.

Knowing that if REM sleep (and dreaming) is suppressed it rebounds, I wondered if my volunteers who had had a couple of hours of drug-induced hallucination experiences during the day would show less "need" to dream the following night. It was a naïve study, not at all well controlled. I did not take into account the amount of brain wave disruption that a hallucinogenic drug would cause in the brains of the sleeping subjects. I found it hard to identify what stage of sleep these normal volunteers were in from their sleep recordings. Their brain waves looked almost as if all stages of sleep were occurring simultaneously. From this point of view, the drug-induced dreaming study was something of a bust. I did collect the subjects' normal dream reports a few nights later when the drug wore off, but more importantly, on the bright side, this study did get me started on the question of why we dream so much and with such great regularity. Perhaps long ago dreaming had a survival purpose, rather like home movies, to keep us entertained and out of harm's way when the sun goes down. If this is true, dreams could be considered a vestigial remnant of our evolutionary past. If so, why then does dreaming persist with such insistence in this day and age? Does it have another purpose, one that is still mysterious to us?

Part of the excitement of working nights in those early days was the opportunity for a psychologist to get a closer look at the mental activity that Freud

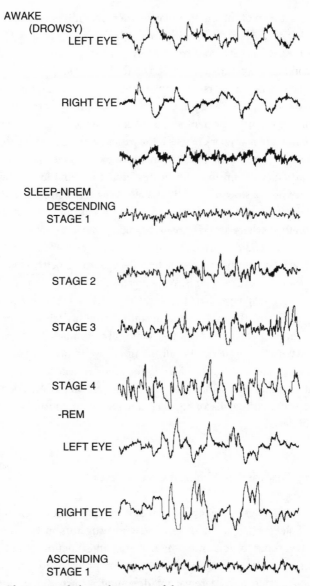

AWAKE
(DROWSY)
    LEFT EYE

RIGHT EYE

SLEEP-NREM
DESCENDING
STAGE 1

STAGE 2

STAGE 3

STAGE 4

-REM

LEFT EYE

RIGHT EYE

ASCENDING
STAGE 1

FIGURE 1.1 Electroencephalographic stages of sleep

believed was crucial to uncovering the motives behind our self-defeating
waking behaviors. Of course, Freud worked from an unrepresentative sample
of persons, analyzing the dreams of patients who were mostly members of the
middle class and who were in some emotional trouble. Although he may not
have known it at the time, he also had a very limited sample of dreams to interpret. We now know that usually, while sleeping at home, we remember at best

only the last dream of the night, and even then only if it is vivid in imagery or particularly rich in feelings. This was established in a 1963 study by Carl Meier, and since then it has been confirmed many times over. Trying to understand a patient's complex psychological makeup on the basis of such a restricted sample is rather like trying to understand a joke simply from hearing the punch line.

Freud did not see this as a problem. He trusted that if a dream was remembered at all, it must be important. In his psychoanalytic treatment, it might take months or more of teamwork between the patient and analyst to trace the many associations, to unravel the multiple memory pathways leading to the reason for this particular dream to occur at this particular time in the patient's life. This was not only a slow process, it was also very expensive. One idea behind sleep and dream research when I began my work was that, with the help of the sleep laboratory, where several dreams could be retrieved every night from a normal adult, we could shorten the time it took to uncover their meaning. The very number of dreams we were able to collect gave us a better chance of identifying repeating dream elements. Were dreams the Rosetta stone written in the mind's memory language? Skeptics argue even today that there is no hidden meaning in dreams themselves; the meanings are only what we project onto what are, in fact, just random neurologically stimulated fragments from memory. After all, people do this all the time—we impose organization onto ambiguous perceptions; we see a Man in the Moon or witches in ink blots. That argument, maintained by Allan Hobson and Robert McCarley, a pair of distinguished neuroscientists, discouraged research on dreaming and its funding for a couple of decades.

How Sleep Disorders Revitalized Dream Research

During the dark days of the 1970s and 1980s, funding for research into the psychology of sleep dried up, and only a few investigators in the United States continued working to determine the meaning and function of dreams. I was one, and Ernest Hartmann was another. It was Ernest who, costumed as an Archbishop during a conference on dreaming, crowned me as Queen of Dreams. Sleep research did not cease entirely at this time, but increasingly became basic research examining the sleep in other species: reptiles, birds, and dolphins, as well as the usual cats, rats, and mice. These animals had a plug surgically implanted through their skulls, so that fine wires could be inserted into brain cells to record their electrical activity in various locations during sleep. Sleep research took on some strange appearances. Once, while visiting a colleague at the University of Chicago sleep lab, which was housed in an old walk-up former residence, I stepped into the bathroom and to my surprise met an implanted alligator observing me from the bath tub.

From these early studies grew an understanding of how the sleeping brain has evolved, which nonhumans sleep and which do not (only rest), which have REM sleep and which only NREM, which sleep with one brain hemisphere at a time while the other stays awake, the mechanisms in various species that turn NREM and REM sleep on and off, and the brain pathways and neurotransmitters involved in stimulating them. We were learning more about the when, where, and how of sleep, but not the *why*. That was the question that kept me going.

During this period, the public became impatient with sleep scientists. After TV appearances during which I would talk about sleep and dreams, hosts would typically ask me when we would be able to address the *practical* problems of sleep. People often called my sleep lab asking for help with their insomnia or jet lag or what to do about their sleepwalking child. Why did they have abrupt "sleep attacks" during the day when they got excited, and could I please tell them what to do about their husband's snoring? Tentatively, sleep research began to shift from studying normal sleepers to examining those with disordered sleep. By the mid 1970s, this became an organized clinical specialty, complete with a formal board examination that had to be passed before one could be approved for treating patients complaining of a sleep disorder. Sleep laboratories also had to be accredited as properly staffed and equipped to carry out diagnostic sleep studies safely.

Wanting to broaden my sleep research to work with patients, I left my teaching job and accepted a position at Rush University Medical Center as Chairman of the Department of Psychology. As part of my negotiations for the job, I met with the austere president of that institution and asked for the space and equipment necessary for opening a sleep disorder service. He leaned forward in his high-backed executive chair, and with his steely blue eyes looked hard into mine and asked "What's that?" At the time, no hospital in the entire state offered clinical services for patients with sleep difficulties. There were only a few anywhere in the country. No wonder he was skeptical.

I got my new five-bed laboratory, with four beds for diagnostic studies of patients and one for research; including a bathroom—for human use only. That was the start of a 30-year stretch during which I wore two hats, or rather coats—a white one when with patients and street clothes for research. By that time, studies conducted around the world had confirmed a set of basic facts about sleep and the unique mental activity going on within it. I will give a short summary description of basic sleep for those readers who may not be familiar with this language.

All humans have regular cycles of REM sleep, even before birth. Newborns spend 50% of their sleep in an active REM-like state. Of course, sleeping babes cannot tell us if they are dreaming—not until they can talk. What is all that REM about in the infant? The speculation is that this active type of sleep in the young stimulates neurons in the brain to grow and to form the networks of connections needed to carry information. After all, the random rapid brain waves of REM sleep do closely resemble those characteristic of waking, when we are attending to the external world.

When we shut our eyes to external stimulation, random rapid brain waves (called "lvf," for low-voltage fast) begin to slow down as we drift off into sleep. These waves progressively slow into what is called Stage 1 sleep. This is the transition from waking into the first of the four stages of NREM sleep. Stage 1 is usually very brief and is followed by Stage 2, identified by two signature waves called *K complexes* and *sleep spindles*. Most of our adult sleep is in Stage 2, and it occupies about 50% of a normal night. The K complexes appear to be responses to either external stimuli like a noise or to some internal stimulus we cannot observe. The sleep spindles may be indicators of some mental activity from waking being reactivated in sleep. This hunch is based on animal recordings during sleep that show increased spindling following new learning trials. Stage 2 next gives way to Stage 3 sleep, with the high slow waves of *delta sleep* mixed in with some remaining Stage 2 activity. When these Stage 2 signs are gone and only the large slow waves of delta sleep take over, this is then called Stage 4, our deepest sleep. Stages 3 and 4 together are called slow-wave sleep (SWS). This SWS should occupy about 20% of the sleep of normal adults. The first SWS episode is usually the longest of the night, and these episodes become shorter each time this sleep reoccurs. By the second half of the night, SWS is typically gone. At the end of the first Stage 4 period there is a lightening of sleep back through Stages 3, then 2, before suddenly the monitors recording the activity of the chin muscles abruptly drop to a flat line, indicating REM is about to begin (Fig. 1.2). This is followed by the eyes beginning to move rapidly. The EEG brain waves of REM are in Stage 1 sleep but, unlike the sleep-onset period of Stage 1 sleep, there is in addition a distinctive loss of muscle tone and rapid synchronous movements of the eyes. The first REM period is brief, usually only 10 minutes or less. The cycling between NREM and REM repeats about every 90 minutes, with each REM period longer than the one before. Together, REM sleep totals to about 25% of the night's sleep.

This alternation of the two types of sleep, the slow then the rapid, the NREM and the REM, throughout the night, suggests some useful division of labor between the two. The large amount of REM sleep during infancy drops by about

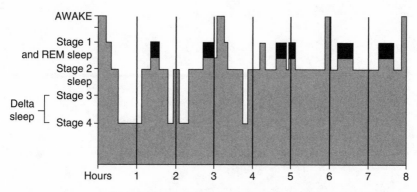

Stage 1 sleep and REM sleep are graphed on the same level
because their EEG patterns are very similar.

FIGURE 1.2 Typical sleep pattern of a young human adult

half, from 50% to 25%, by the time a baby has turned into a 1-year-old child. The brain continues to sprout new connections throughout life as we learn and save our new experiences in memory, but the original big wiring job that enables us to rapidly absorb information from the world we are born into and to which we must learn how to respond, is laid down in that first year. There is no question that REM sleep plays an important role in this process.

What about dreams? When, how, and why do they develop? After all, although dreaming and REM coincide, they are not the same thing. Here, the research with animals is no help (even though many dog owners are sure that their pet does dream). At times, dogs appear to be imagining chasing squirrels or rabbits; this is most apparent when they lay limply asleep, making little whining noises while twitching their paws, and flickering movements of their eyes are visible under their closed lids. Unfortunately, we cannot verify what they are experiencing by asking them to share it with us. We can only measure their brain activity and hypothesize from there. Children, fortunately, do learn to talk, and can talk about what is happening in their minds while sleeping, so let's look next at how our dream lives begin.

Collecting Dreams: Watching the | 2
Sleeping Mind

Children begin by loving their parents. After a time they
judge them. Rarely if ever do they forgive them.

—Oscar Wilde, *A Woman of No Importance*

For the most part, parents are only aware that their children are dreaming
when they wake from a nightmare and need to be calmed down before they
can get back to sleep. But in fact children experience a good deal of rapid eye
movement (REM) sleep before they have the language skills to tell us whether
anything like a dream is happening. This leaves parents with very few options,
the most popular being turning on the light to prove to the child that he or she
is safe at home, then giving them a warm hug while denying that there are
witches or other scary creatures hiding in the closet. When children do have
enough language to tell us what had been going on during sleep, we have a
chance to hear what has been frightening them and to do some educating on
the spot about the source of dreams. My own technique when my children were
small was to encourage them to tell me what they were experiencing and to
listen carefully; I would praise their reports, saying something like, "That was
an interesting story you were telling yourself. I wonder why you were telling
that one?" The message is, "It is your story. You made it up, and we can figure it

out together." This usually consoles children, and more important, it puts them in charge. A bad dream then is not something being done *to* them, but something of their own making. The second part of the message, "I wonder why you were telling that one?," challenges children to think about what strongly felt waking experiences they remember and to learn to understand the connection between these and their dreams.

David Foulkes, a psychologist and father of sons, explains in the first few pages of his classic 1982 book *Children's Dreams* why he undertook his landmark longitudinal study of the dreams of a group of children he recorded over several years. In part, he blames Freud. Freud's book *The Interpretation of Dreams* had profound influence on the thinking of developmental psychologists at the time. Foulkes states that he was irked by statements these professionals would make about children's dreams based on Freud's theories—which had never been formally tested. He was especially irritated by those developmental experts who theorized that "underneath the superficial placidity of much of a child's waking behavior lies a set of animalistic impulses and egotistical wishes that bode ill for the child's prospects for a harmonious social adaptation and, ultimately for our own as well, because inside each of us there also lies this same infantile irrationality (p.6)." Foulkes is a scientist, and as far as he was concerned, this grim conception of human behavior had no proven basis in fact. He set out to correct this by finding out just how dreams actually develop from year to year, starting when children are very young. By testing the children's waking mental abilities and collecting their dreams at night, Foulkes expected that he would be able to obtain evidence that changes in children's cognitive abilities to express themselves evolve systematically, and to find out whether dreams do have some specific unique characteristics and functions.

Foulkes worked with two groups of children, a younger group of 3- or 4-year-olds and an older group of 9- or 10-year-olds. He followed these children over a 5-year period, conducting sleep studies on them every few weeks. In this way, Foulkes covered the age span from 3 to 15. This was a truly heroic endeavor, as he did all of the night recordings by himself. Each child slept in the laboratory eight to ten times every year. Foulkes was there every night, and conducted all the awakenings from the children's REM sleep to ask about their dreams. That added up to a total of 1,347 sleepless nights for him. After the many nights spent recording these children's dreams, Foulkes was in for a shock when he began his systematic examination of the data. Only 27% of the times he awakened his preschoolers during their REM sleep did they actually tell him a dream. Once he got over this surprise, he reasoned that their reports were probably few because these children were not yet capable of sophisticated "image representation and narrative organization." These skills, he hypothesized, develop slowly in early childhood, and had not yet "reached that critical mass" required for describing a dream. When the younger children did tell him their dreams, they were notably short, usually consisting of only a single sentence, with no action and no well-constructed plot. Foulkes noted too that the main characters were more often animals than humans.

In general, my own experiences studying children in the sleep lab mirror Foulkes', although when a child could not tell me a dream, I supplied paper and crayons and asked the child to draw it. In one of those drawings, a scary-looking monster with a large head and wide open mouth showing sharp teeth hovers over the bed of the small stick figure of a child (Fig. 2.1). This was drawn by a 3-year-old. It did not need a story; it was eloquent enough all by itself. Clearly, this child was fully capable of representing her REM experience in an image, but did not yet have the verbal skills to turn it into a dream report. What prompted that dream? I suspect it was a response to something that had happened the evening before. She was dawdling, prolonging getting ready for a night in our lab. Her normally even-tempered mother lost her cool, and suddenly yelled at her, momentarily turning into a scary, big-mouthed monster.

Foulkes sums up his conclusions about the dreams of his 3- to 5-year-old group rather churlishly. He blames the low frequency of dream reports on their cognitive immaturity, referring to the children as "constrained and impoverished, defective in inventiveness."

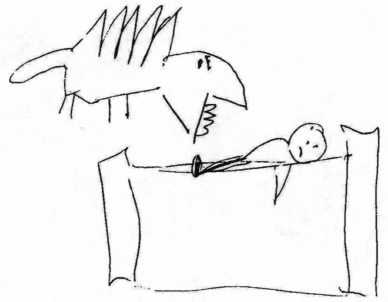

FIGURE 2.1 Dream drawing of a 3-year-old girl

When the children were 5 to 7 years old, their dream reports were longer, although the frequency of dreams reported was not much higher. The proportion of times these children remembered a dream when awakened from REM sleep was just 31%. This is still a long way from the report rate of adults, who can be counted on to tell a dream 85% of the time when they are interrupted while in a REM sleep interval. Animal characters were still common in the 5- to 7-year-old children's dreams—more so in boys than in girls, and more often in boys who were socially immature and were having "impulse control problems in their waking behavior." (This last bit is most interesting, as it implies that personality and/or behavior can be predicted, at least in part, by the content of a child's dreams.) Foulkes tentatively suggested that the animal dreams of children at this age may reflect their real-life conflicts about controlling their impulsiveness. In this age group, there were still very few dreams with a self character and very few with any mention of emotion.

When the children were studied at the next age level of 7 to 9 years old, there were fewer animal characters and more humans, and more of these were family members. Figures 2.2 and 2.3 are dream drawings by an 8-year-old girl who tells a complicated story of relations with her mother and sister, and in Figures 2.4 and 2.5, she writes her own dream and an interpretation of her dream. It is notable that she is the daughter of a psychologist (she is not

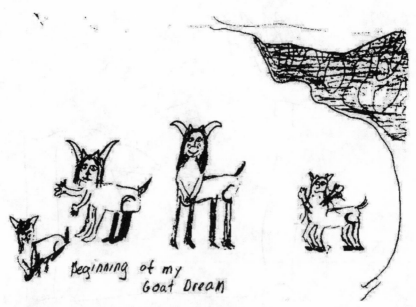

Beginning of my
Goat Dream

FIGURE 2.2 Dream drawings of an 8-year-old girl

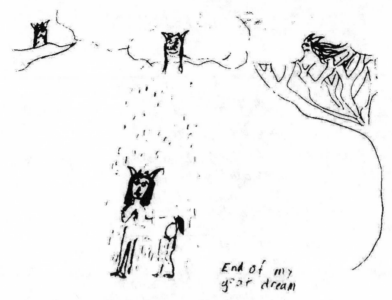

End of my
year dream

FIGURE 2.3 Dream drawings of an 8-year-old girl

My Dream

My mom, my sisters, & I were
all goats. We lived happily.
One day I got mad at
them & I killed them.
My mom was a goddess,
I was on earth starving
for I was still a
baby & needed milk.
My mom felt sorry
for me & made it
rain warm milk
so I wouldn't starve.

FIGURE 2.4 An 8-year-old's dream

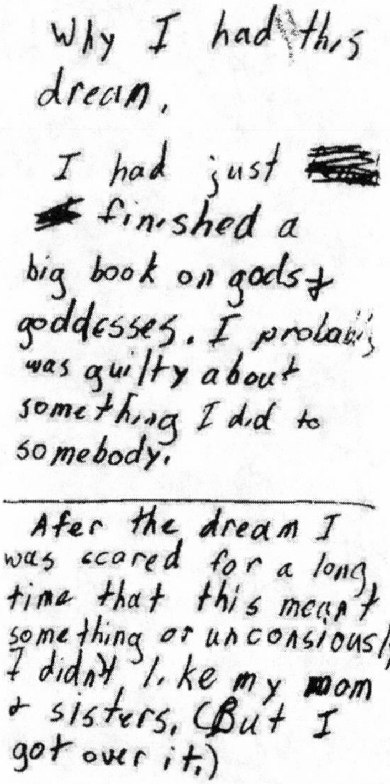

> Why I had this dream,
>
> I had just ~~finished~~ finished a big book on gods + goddesses. I probably was guilty about something I did to somebody.
>
> ___
>
> After the dream I was scared for a long time that this meant something or unconsiously I didn't like my mom + sisters. (But I got over it.)

FIGURE 2.5 An 8-year-old's written interpretations of her dream

my daughter). Girls at this age were found to have more male adult strangers in their dreams. (When I was about 6 or 7 years old, I recall dreaming of a male stranger; he remained a lifetime member of my dream stock company. He shows up in a dream whenever I need reminding of the threat he represents to my self image. I will report this dream in Chapter 9, along with my method for understanding how it is constructed and why.)

Foulkes' older group of children, those 11 to 13 years of age, reported dreams more frequently—the recall rate jumps then to 66%. Once again, the higher rate was more characteristic of children who were more verbally imaginative and assertive while awake. Family characters are now less frequent. Particularly interesting was the finding that there were fewer dreams featuring a mother character. Foulkes states that the maternal family value structure is less important for both boys and girls at this age, and that the home is less often the setting of their dreams. At this age, dreams are beginning to show a trend toward a psychological readiness to separate from home and to establish independence from the mother—to imagine leaving childhood behind. Dreams seem to be illustrating the children's process of growing up.

In his book, Foulkes concluded that his study cast serious doubt on the Freudian theory that regular every-night experiencing of dreams serves to regulate the basic drives, particularly those most unacceptable, of sex and aggression, which were only somewhat tamed in waking expression by the child's increasing conformity to social norms. Again in theory, dreams were the venue in which these drives could find indirect expression, helping to keep the peace by preventing their intruding into awareness. Foulkes did leave room for the possibility that the sleep itself, the unique REM state, may be involved in regulating these drives, but that what is actually dreamed does not. He emphasized that the dream story is closely related to these children's waking level of cognitive and symbolic development, rather than to their emotional or motivational states, agreeing with Calvin Hall, a senior psychologist and dream researcher who concluded from his own work that dreams reveal how we think about ourselves, and our relations to significant others and the world about us. Foulkes closed his book with words that emphasize this conception: "In children's dreams we find what and how children think about themselves. These ideas, about who we are, the self, whether we are aware of them consciously in wakefulness or not, are the key component of the programmatic regulation we exercise over our behavior." That is a serious statement, and one I think is basically true, but it does not clearly follow from his findings, which I believe were biased by the method he used to collect the dreams. By requiring the children to describe their experience verbally, Foulkes over-emphasized the cognitive and under-represented the emotional aspect of dreams, which children's dream drawings capture most vividly.

Dreams of Adults

Many adults also find dream reporting in the laboratory to be a difficult task. Being awakened abruptly and asked to translate fleeting visual images into verbal descriptions that an investigator can understand is not only hard on the sleeper; it has frequently left me, as the experimenter, feeling like the teacher in a "Peanuts" cartoon. In one strip, we see a little girl sitting at her desk saying, "Sorry Ma'am. I was asleep and I dreamed I was sleeping, but in the dream where I was sleeping I dreamed I was awake. Then in the dream where I was awake I fell asleep and in the dream where I was sleeping I heard your voice and woke up. Anyway I think that was how it was. Did you ask me a question? Please don't cry, Ma'am."

The translation problem from visual to verbal is still a hurdle for many sleep study volunteers, but because their verbal skills are more developed, adults' dreams are somewhat easier to follow than are those of young children. Further complicating dream collection is the added problem of the influence of the sleeper's relationship to the experimenter, and sleepers' motivations for cooperating in the study. Some sleepers are more interested in getting back to sleep as quickly as possible than they are in providing a full dream report. As a result, their reports may be short and under-represented. Other sleepers may wish to please the experimenter by providing a rich report, going on and on, making many revisions to their dream story. They may add bits to extend the story or double back to revise their report. In my lab, we try to avoid this variability in the length of the time the person stays awake because of its effect on the report. We keep the time awake short and relatively constant, allowing only a 3- to 5-minute window for collecting the remembered dream. To implement this, we encourage the short reporters by asking, "Anything else?" and limit the long reporters by thanking them and urging them to get back to sleep, promising we will wake them again later on.

Fred Snyder, a psychiatrist who was the chief of the Clinical Psychobiology Laboratory at the National Institute of Mental Health, undertook a detailed study of the dreams of young adults. He picks up with the age group following where Foulkes left off. Snyder was well aware of all the difficulties of obtaining dream reports in the laboratory. He put it this way in an often-quoted chapter summarizing his work in 1970: "Our approach is probably as close as we can get to dreaming consciousness, at least until technical ingenuity provides a means of reproducing the conscious perception of the dreamer as it occurs." All of us who depend on the laboratory method to investigate dreams share the fantasy that some day we will have monitors capable of transmitting not just electronic signals, but the images themselves as they are being experienced by the sleeper. Such technology might project dream images onto a screen, so that researchers could watch the dream as it unfolds. This idea is itself still just a dream, of course. The laboratory method of dream collecting ensures that we get many samples of the night's mental experiences, but these are not pure samples. One of the worst "contaminants" in dream research comes from our need to awaken subjects for reports throughout the night. Studies that have looked at these reports in search of continuity of a particular theme within one night must acknowledge that by making the dreamer consciously aware of the contents of the first dream by awakening and asking for a report, they may influence in some the sleeper's dream trajectory as it enters into the next REM period. In this way, the laboratory method may be inducing the very continuity we are testing. Dream work is full of many such booby-traps.

To find out what adults were dreaming, Snyder turned to a data bank of 635 dreams he had collected over 250 nights. These were recorded from a sample of mostly middle-class college students with diverse backgrounds. His purpose in undertaking this review was just to see what he would find. This is markedly different from the work done by Foulkes, who was on a mission to refute the psychoanalytic layer-cake model of the mind. But, surprisingly, Snyder came to a conclusion similar to that of Foulkes. "Dreaming consciousness," he states, "is a remarkably faithful replica of waking life." His sleepers produced no abstract works of art. Instead, "in almost every instance the progression of complex visual imagery described a realistic facsimile of the visual perception of external reality." Every report was animated, and all but a few featured human figures. Most striking was the pervasiveness of the self in these college students' dreams. "The all-important 'I' appeared in 95% of the dreams," but only rarely was the "I" alone. Family members were present in 19% of the dreams, friends and acquaintances in 35%, and in 46%, the others were unknowns. There were very few popular or cult figures. Only rarely did a president or movie star appear. Even the dreamed animals were not exotic creatures, but mostly domestic pets. What were all of those dreamed people doing? Mostly they were talking. Seventy-six percent of the dreams included some auditory imagery, most often speech, but music might also be playing, or dogs barking, or rain falling. Snyder made another interesting observation: that, in addition to what is happening in the foreground, there is also a more or less "continuous background accompaniment of reflections and attitudes, as well as clear evidence at times of inferential thinking, remembering, deciding, feelings of volition and, of course, emotion."

Tracking emotion in dream reports has given sleep researchers a good deal of trouble. The problem is that emotion is often implicit in the narrative rather than explicitly named. It is easy to think we know which emotion *should* be appropriate within the circumstances of a dream story, but we are frequently wrong. Snyder found feelings were only mentioned spontaneously in a third of the dreams. When they were explicit, they were more often unpleasant than pleasant, with a 2:1 ratio. Fear, anxiety, and anger were the most common negative emotions present in dreams, whereas on the pleasant side, "friendliness" was number one. Primitive emotions—those that many Freudians might expect to find—were conspicuously absent. Nevertheless, Snyder suggested that Freud might speculate that the paucity of emotion in laboratory dreams could be the result of a "heightening of the forces of censorship during sleep," especially when the dreamer knows they must report what is going on to an experimenter who may be an authority figure. (I know I had this effect when my students were the volunteer sleepers and I was both the experimenter and their professor.) Ultimately, though, Snyder decided that the blandness of dreams as told in the laboratory is simply the true reflection of our everyday lives. He argued in his chapter "The Phenomenology of Dreaming" that the exciting dreams we remember at home are the rare dramatic ones.

There is evidence to the contrary. Ample research supports that dreams are longer, more complex in structure and more emotion-filled at the end of the night than they are in the beginning, and since we are more likely to remember the dream that we are experiencing just as we wake up, we are likely to best remember the wildest one of the night. This was confirmed as early as 1968, in a study by Carl Meier, and the findings have been replicated frequently since. Studies comparing dreams collected in the privacy of the home to those told to an experimenter in a lab have shown that home dreams are "juicier." So compelling is the contrast that equipment has been developed to help sleep researchers collect dream reports from people sleeping at home. In one of these, a lightweight electrode is placed on an eye lid and a buzzer is programmed to wake the sleeper when a preset number of rapid eye movements occur. At that point, a voice-activated tape recorder turns on so that the dreamer can give their report and preserve it without an experimenter being involved. Home dreams collected in this way are more emotional, with more sex and aggression than those reported by the same person in a laboratory. It seems clear that laboratory conditions produce a dampening effect on the reports and probably also on the very construction of the dreams themselves. Those sleep researchers who want to test some hypothesis about the function of dreaming (do they express forbidden motives?) must recognize that they need to control for the laboratory effect or find another way to test this hypothesis.

Brain Imaging in Sleep

Neither Foulkes' views on children's dreams, nor Snyder's on the dreams of young adults, were likely to convince a granting agency that further studies of dreams held much promise of breakthroughs in understanding the mind. It would take another technical advance to stimulate further dream research, and brain imaging during sleep was one of these next steps. Brain imaging allowed researchers to pinpoint those areas of the brain that are more and less active in sleep than they are in waking, and to compare the brain scans of normal sleepers to those with some known sleep or psychiatric diagnosis. The advent of sophisticated imaging techniques such as positron emission tomography (PET) scans and functional magnetic resonance imaging (fMRI) just might provide the kind of hard evidence needed to legitimatize the premise that something different happens in the brain during sleep and in dreaming than we are able to observe in the waking state. This "something" turned out to be not less activity in all areas, as might have been expected, but more in some. In fact, brain scans show different patterns of activation and deactivation within the brain during the three states we cycle through during each 24 hours: waking, non-REM (NREM), and REM sleep. During REM, there is less activity in the prefrontal cortex (the seat of the so-called executive functions of logical thinking, judging, decision making, and self-reflecting) and more in the sensory association areas, and those sites associated with emotion (the limbic and paralimbic areas). In those who are mentally healthy, these areas of the brain light up, showing much higher activity during REM than is present during waking. This suggests that, in REM sleep, we are seeing and hearing things that are not logical but probably have emotional associations, and confirms what we thought was the nature of dreaming from listening to many sleepers' REM reports. The brain scans give these conclusions the weight of technological support.

How about those with sleep troubles? We now have studies examining the differences between patients diagnosed with various sleep and psychiatric disorders and healthy control subjects. Major depression is one illness that has yielded interesting results, and I will review these in Chapter 4. As for sleepwalking, it has been difficult to conduct a brain imaging study of a sleepwalker in action because this is not an every-night occurrence, and without an overt attempt to walk, a typical sleep recording itself does not reveal any specific differences from those of matched nonwalkers. So far, there has been just one study of a sleepwalker while sleepwalking, published in 2000. The subject was a 16-year-old male who frequently walked in sleep, just as he had done since childhood. He was being recorded for a standard sleep study called a polysomnogram (PSG), meaning that many monitors were recording bodily functions as well as his brain waves. These were recorded by electroencephalography (EEG), the eye movements by oculograms, heart rate by electrocardiogram (EKG), and by electrodes placed on other areas of the body to record muscle tone at the chin and movement in the legs. Respiratory effort and blood oxygen saturation levels are also typically included in a standard study.

The sleepwalker not only had a known history of sleepwalking, but so did his maternal grandmother, mother, and younger brother. It was clear that he had inherited a genetic flaw in the motor control system of sleep, one that made him vulnerable to getting up and walking about when he should have been quietly sleeping. During his first night of laboratory study he did not perform, he just slept all night. On the second night, however, he was asleep for less than an hour and was deep into his NREM Stages 3 and 4, slow wave sleep (SWS), when he abruptly sat up, got out of bed looking scared, and mumbled something unintelligible. That happened at 11:13 P.M. Twenty-four seconds later, he was injected with a dye that would reveal what was happening in his brain, and a single-photon emission computed tomography (SPECT) study was performed. His brain scan was then compared to those of non-sleepwalkers at the same amount of time from sleep onset. The authors of this study state that the test showed the sleepwalker had "dissociation between motor arousal and mental sleep." The cerebral blood flow was 25% higher in the brain regions known as the cingulate cortex and the thalamus than is seen in normal sleepers, while at the same time there was less activity in the frontoparietal associative cortices. The authors suggest that these patterns are consistent with a state of emotional and motor arousal along with a lack of self-awareness, insight, and recall. That supports a lot of what we had speculated was going on in the brain when sleepwalking events happen.

This single but important look at the brain activity of a sleepwalker during an episode confirmed that he was emotionally aroused and his body active, while at the same time the higher mental processes of judgment, rational thought, self-reflection, and memory were still asleep. These patients seem to be caught in a mixed, in-between state; both brain scan and behavior suggest they are partly awake and partly asleep. This study also confirms that sleepwalking begins while the sleeper is in SWS. This was first established by Roger Broughton, a neurologist who showed that sleepwalking is not related to dreaming. But every sleep-related answer introduces another question: What was going on in the sleepwalker's mind then that caused him to get up looking scared? To a casual observer, it might seem he was having a bad dream, or remembering one—but both the brain scan and sleep study indicated he was not. The authors of the study did not tell us what usually happened when he sleepwalked at home, where his activity would not be restricted by the monitors he was required to wear in the lab study. Nor did they tell us what the young man was talking about before the study started, perhaps while the technician was getting the electrodes attached—this could have influenced his behavior while asleep. If we knew more about what was on his mind before he went to sleep, we might have found some clues to understanding his motivation for the walk, and why he looked so scared.

Fear has been the most common answer sleepwalkers give when asked what they remember after having sat up abruptly in our lab, looking panicky. One man reported that this fear was accompanied by the image of a very large black spider on the clean white wall facing his bed. He stared at it intently while the technician tried to ask him what was going on. It took him several minutes to come out of this confused state, to realize where he was, and return to sleep. At this point, brain imaging in sleep is rather a blunt instrument in its contribution to our understanding of how the mind is working on its own in sleep, but it does reveal differences between patient groups and confirms some of our hunches.

We know a good deal from what normal sleepers tell us of their experiences during the time of night associated with sleepwalking, the first hour of NREM sleep—simply by waking them in the laboratory. But these reports are not as consistent as those we retrieve from REM sleep. From REM awakenings, we hear a story made up of loosely connected sensory images, in which, as Fred Snyder put it, the all important "I" is usually interacting with others. What is more, the sleeper believes what he is dreaming is the truth. In other words, we are hallucinating while asleep. Luckily, this state is quickly reversible when we wake up and return to reality. When awakened from their first NREM SWS, sleepers tell us most often that "nothing at all" has been going on, or just that "I was sleeping," just before we asked for a report. But some give a short statement that sounds very different from the image-rich narratives we call dreams. "I was thinking about . . . " or "I was wondering if . . . " is the way these are often phrased. Also the sleeper knows these are thoughts going on in their own minds and not something they believe to be really happening. As I hinted earlier, there is a third kind of report from NREM awakenings that does sound more dreamlike. These are more often single images not connected by a story line. Mostly they occur during the first few minutes of very light NREM sleep, the transitional sleep from waking into Stages 1 and 2. They are of use to us now in tracking what is being carried forward from waking into the first few minutes of sleep.

The Benefit of NREM and REM Cooperation

In the last few years, there has been a revival of interest in the possible role of sleep in problem solving and in preserving newly learned skills in memory so that performance of that skill is improved the next day. In short, "sleeping on it" is wise advice. Think back to "take two aspirins and call me in the morning." Want to improve your golf stroke? Concentrate on it before sleeping. An interval of sleep has been proven to bestow a real benefit for both laboratory animals and humans when they are tested on many different types of newly learned tasks. You will remember more items or make fewer mistakes if you have had a period of sleep between learning something new and the test of your ability to recall it later than you would if you spent the same amount of time awake. Once these positive results began to be published, this line of research accelerated. How much sleep is needed to produce this positive effect? Will a short nap help, or must the interval be equal to a full night's sleep? What kind of sleep does the trick, REM sleep or NREM? If it is NREM, is it the slow waves of Stages 3 and 4, or the lighter Stage 2 sleep with sleep spindles? All have been studied and "all won prizes," as Louis Carroll might say.

Most investigators agree with the overall conclusion that one of the ways that sleep works is by enhancing the memory of important bits of new information and clearing out unnecessary or competing bits, and then passing the good bits on to be integrated into existing memory circuits. This happens in two steps. The first is in early NREM sleep when the brain circuits that were active while we were learning something new, a motor skill, say, or a new language, are reactivated and stay active until REM sleep occurs. In REM sleep, these new bits of information are then matched to older related memories already stored in long-term memory networks. This causes the new learning to stick (to be consolidated) and to remain accessible for when we need it later in waking.

Here are a few examples of how this works. How do rats remember the way through a maze or the details of some other new environment? While they explore new territory, rats are building a spatial map in memory. The new sensory information they receive through their paws and whiskers as they find their way through the floor and walls of a maze activates special "place cells" in the brain area known as the hippocampus. When the animal sleeps, these place cells are reactivated, a sign that memory is being formed and consolidated. This is detected by recording the activity from electrode arrays placed into brain cells. Of course, we cannot place electrodes deep into brain cells of humans for research purposes. But we do know a little from direct probing of brain cell activity in patients who are undergoing brain surgeries to relieve intractable seizures, and who gave their consent for this procedure. Such patients are kept awake, so that they can report their experience while electrodes probe to find the exact location of the seizure activity, thereby helping the neurosurgeon avoid removing any healthy tissue.

We can see the same kind of sleep-related memory formation process in humans by pasting small electrodes onto the surface of the face near the outer edge of each eye. These measure the rapid eye movements that take place during each REM period, and they show a marked increase when we have been concentrating on learning something new. It is not the amount of time in REM sleep that increases during memory formation, but how active are the eyes close to the time during which we are immersed in mastering something new.

Carlyle Smith, a Canadian psychologist, studied his students' sleep and counted their REM eye movements just after they had been studying hard for their mid-term exams. He then brought the students back to the lab during their summer vacation 6 months later, monitoring their sleep again. This time, the students' eye movement counts were much lower. Interestingly, the higher-achieving the student, the bigger the difference in eye movement counts between the time of heavy learning and their time off. Those who were lower achieving had less of a difference in their eye movement scores. The conclusion was that the smarter students were storing more information during sleep when they were actively studying hard than were the low-achieving students. Smith then looked into what effect alcohol before sleep would have on this memory consolidation process. He found that it interfered with memory formation, reducing the number of rapid eye movements.

If these eye movements represent the reactivation during sleep of the scanning we do of new visual information, like the movements of the eyes as they scan across a page while we read, would they also show an increase with other kinds of nonverbal learning? It seems that the answer is yes; results similar to Smith's were found in volunteers learning Morse code. Those who had the highest number of rapid eye movements in their REM sleep following a 90-minute learning session just before sleeping in the lab had the highest scores on a Morse code test given the next day.

The next logical step is to investigate how new information crosses over from waking into sleep, so that it can be consolidated later when the active sleep of REM takes place. Surely we do not need to save *everything* that happens each day. What information is selected, why, and how? Now we are getting to the heart of the matter. To learn more about this process, we must move back, from focusing on what happens in REM sleep and whether dreams contribute to this memory process, to examining what happens at the very beginning of sleep. That is the magical moment when we shift from being aware and in charge to a state in which we blank out, and some other process takes over. Decision-making is no longer under our conscious control. Research going on now is zeroing in on that transition point, the first minutes of sleep onset, to look into what is on our minds at that moment and how the brain transmits this from NREM to REM sleep, so that we may hold onto it in memory for subsequent waking use.

As early as the 1950s and '60s, when sleep research was young, many investigators woke their subjects during the NREM cycles as a control procedure for REM awakenings. This allowed us to study whether dreams were confined to REM sleep or whether this hallucinatory type of mental behavior depends on the time of night. Would reports from both NREM and REM sleep at the end of the night be "dreamier" than those from early in the night? These studies confirmed that reports from REM are generally of a different order from the style of those going on during most of NREM sleep for most people. There are some exceptions to this rule, but for the most part the spontaneous thinking in NREM tends to be more logical and linear: "I was wondering when I would get paid for this study," while in REM the reports are more perceptual and emotional: "I was escaping from something, and was spreading ketchup on pieces of my clothing and hanging them on branches to make my pursuers think I was injured."

In the new studies investigating what carries forward from waking into sleep, volunteers are given tasks that require them to work hard, focusing for hours at a time. They then are awakened within the first few minutes of sleep and asked what they remember of their thoughts before being woken. Can we catch some remnants of the day's effort and follow the progress of memory formation and consolidation across the hours of sleep? At first, the results were slim. Robert Stickgold, a sleep researcher at Harvard, has been publishing on a series of these studies, which started in 1998. He first had volunteers play the video game Tetris 2 or 3 hours a day for 3 days before waking them and asking them to report what they were aware of within the first 3 minutes of sleep. Would they see images from the game? Sixty-four percent of the volunteers did report seeing the Tetris tiles fall into place, but they also reported much more that was going on in their minds at the time. Mostly what the volunteers were experiencing were private thoughts, not images, about their own concerns.

Next, Stickgold tried having his volunteers spend time on virtual skiing using Alpine Racer II. This involved movement and visual input, as well as coordination of the two. Again he interrupted the first few minutes of sleep to ask what was on the volunteers' minds. His aim was to test whether specific images from the game continue into sleep and, if they did, whether they were in some way "useful" the next day, perhaps in improving their performance on the game. This time, he also woke the sleepers 2 hours after they fell asleep, so that he could determine whether skiing images survived the transition into sleep, and how these changed as sleep progressed into the second NREM sleep cycle. To test for the "functionality" of such incorporations, he waited until they had had a first REM period and were back into the next period of NREM sleep.

These are early results, but they indicate that what gets our attention while playing these virtual reality games (and, by extension, what gets stored as permanent memory) are those images associated with strong emotion, such as the places in the game where a crash took place. These are the images that were incorporated into the first few minutes of sleep, particularly in those players who had previous real skiing experience. Interestingly, this phenomenon also occurred in control subjects. These were onlookers who observed the players as they actively worked at mastering the game, and who then also slept in the lab. Those nonparticipant controls who had skied previously also showed some incorporation of skiing images into their first few minutes of sleep. For the Tetris game, the same thing happened; those who had previous experience playing Tetris for fun (before they participated in this study) were the ones who incorporated visual images of the game into their early NREM sleep. In other words, the players who had already stored some memories related to the laboratory task were more likely to preserve new memories obtained during the experiment, especially if these had emotional significance that somehow marked them as important. Without a memory network already in place, the experience of the experimental tasks was typically purged from sleep in favor of the players' own ongoing personal concerns. These trumped the experiment as more important to them.

Promising findings came from waking the players 2 hours after they fell asleep while they were in their second NREM cycle. At that time, mental images that could be identified as being related to the game appeared to have undergone some transformation. One example of this effect Stickgold offers is from the report of a sleeper who, after hours of playing Alpine Racer, reported from the second NREM cycle that "I felt as though I was falling downhill." There was no mention of skiing imagery; falling downhill could apply to many different kinds of activities—in other words, the specific has become the general. Stickgold speculates that the appearance in the first few minutes of sleep of specific images carried over from waking initiates a process that "ultimately leads to the integration of these new experiences into the individual's broader network of (semantic) knowledge." These are very preliminary results, but intriguing nonetheless.

It seems that out of all new experience of a day, what our brains retain and replay in our sleep are those bits which seem familiar, based on previous experience—particularly those that have an emotional charge. These find their way to a place in the memory network where similar experiences are stored. This demonstrates that there is an important interaction between waking and NREM sleep.

We can now begin to answer the question, "Where do we go when we go to sleep?" Clearly, we do not sink into a void, but instead into a mental workshop where emotionally important information is kept active until it is saved in neural networks. When the highly activated REM sleep comes along, perceptual dreams reveal the matching of new information to old, at first in rather simple terms: "I dreamed about my boyfriend but he looked just like an uncle of mine who left his wife." Through the night, from REM to REM, new information is integrated, drawing together more and more remote associations. The dream story line gets stretched into increasingly illogical and bizarre connections. No wonder we wake saying, "I had the craziest dream," or "What was that about?" Proof of the short-term functionality, or usefulness, of this process lies in what happens the next morning. There occurs both down-regulation of negative mood, as we will see in Chapter 4, and improved memory with better performance on newly learned tasks. What I am most interested in as a sleep researcher is the proposition that the long-term effect of healthy sleep is to continuously test and modify those nonconscious habitual schemas that make up our self-system and influence our behavior choices, based on our emotional evaluation of whether the new experience supports or challenges our present self-definition. This is a considerable task for sleep to perform. Let's now test this proposal by seeing what happens when we short-change this important process by sleeping less.

Short Sleep and Its Consequences: Insomnia

Some people require eight hours, nature requires seven.
Nine hours laziness, and wickedness eleven.

—Anonymous

We live in a culture that values speed; fast foods, fast cars, fast service, and fast decisions. All of this takes a toll. Fast food is blamed for the epidemic of obesity, fast cars for motor vehicle accidents, and the wish for fast service and decisions for an increase in the general level of frustration when we are inevitably put on hold. This "hurry up" lifestyle also has an impact on sleep—it has notably shortened the number of hours we as a society devote to it. When sleep experts speak to general audiences, one question they are often asked is, "How can I spend less time sleeping?" Those who ask this question tell us that sleep is a waste of time. Not only is that notion wrong, but the attitude behind it is largely responsible for the increase of several major public health problems.

We now turn to those whose short number of sleep hours is troubling enough for them that they seek professional help. This is not the case for all short sleepers; some manage to live productive lives and make significant contributions to society. These are the ones who occupy the extreme left-hand tail of a normal distribution of average hours of sleep needed to feel rested. Most of us will fall in the middle of that curve, needing between 7 and 9 hours, with an average close to 8. Short sleepers average 5.5 hours. Very few people are truly physiologically and psychologically healthy with only 5 hours of sleep on a nightly basis. Those who, as adults, were 8-hour sleepers but can no longer get that much sleep are in trouble. Some cannot get to sleep without a prolonged struggle, while others get to sleep but wake repeatedly. Then there are those who wake too early and cannot get back to sleep. Insomnia is a useful model to test the contribution of sleep to keeping us healthy in mind and body.

The Costs of Short Sleep

What is the definition of "short sleep"? Sleep experts are reluctant to answer this question by giving a specific number of hours. As noted, there is just too much variability among individuals in the amount of sleep it takes for them to accomplish the "rest and restoration" functions of sleep. When we are getting "enough" sleep, we wake up feeling physically refreshed, in a reasonably good mood, and able to function well throughout the day without undue sleepiness. All of us experience a down time around mid-afternoon, called the "circadian dip," or sometimes known by the more colorful name, "circadian slump." This is when our internal body temperatures drop, bringing on a natural tendency to feel sleepy enough for a midday siesta. If you can get through this without falling asleep at your desk or in your car and then feel all right for the rest of the day, your number of sleep hours is right for you.

Another indicator of how much sleep is enough is the number of hours we sleep when sleep is unscheduled—that is, when we need not wake at a set time, like on weekends and vacations. Since we tend to go to bed later under these circumstances we also tend to sleep later, so it is not the hour at which we wake that makes the difference but how many hours we sleep when we can take our time. If you sleep 2 or 3 hours more on weekend nights than you do during weeknights, you are probably not getting enough sleep on a regular basis. This is what Bill Dement calls running a "sleep debt," and this debt must be paid back by extending your regular sleep schedule or by including some daytime naps.

A trend among American adults is to sleep fewer hours a night during the work week and to play catch-up on the weekends. This is proof that many who report they are short sleepers actually can sleep longer, but do not by choice. According to information about our sleep habits gathered periodically by the Centers for Disease Control and Prevention, the old 8-hour national average per night has dropped to 7. Evidence that this is a real problem can be found in the push to develop new drugs to treat sleep troubles. In addition to new sleeping pills, we now see new "stay awake" pills marketed to help keep us going even longer, to work more hours without experiencing a drop in the quality of our job performance. For those who suffer from a neurological problem such as narcolepsy, one symptom of which is sudden abrupt sleep episodes that come without warning, these medications are a life-altering boon. But for those who are healthy, the cost to our health of working longer hours by sleeping less is not worth the benefit.

Another more alarming trend we see now is the misuse by adolescents and young adults of "stay-awake" prescription medications such as Ritalin, Adderall, and modafinil originally developed to treat attention-deficit hyperactivity disorder (ADHD). More and more frequently these drugs are being used by young people to increase their focused attention. Is this harmful? Yes, if it interferes with the ability to get enough sleep, and for sure if the drug was not prescribed but is "borrowed" from someone else.

Some who sleep 6 or fewer hours argue that this is not by choice but by economic necessity, the result of having to work two jobs. Data show that the use of stay-awake medicine is strongly related to shift work. Daytime sleep is shorter and lighter than nighttime sleep and so less refreshing. Those who report using stay-awake medications point out that there is simply too much to do in a 16-hour day, and that an 8-hour night is a luxury they can no longer afford. The economic need may be real but the price we pay for such a heavy sleep debt should be better understood. It is especially important for physicians to understand the risks involved in aiding their patients to reduce sleep hours with a prescription, and it is up to sleep experts to offer some sensible alternatives.

Evidence that enough sleep is a necessity for both physical and mental health has been accumulating for years. Many studies show the detrimental effects on cats, rats, and healthy human volunteers of reducing the amount of their sleep, sometimes down to zero. The best of the recent experiments using rats was carried out by Allan Rechtschaffen of the University of Chicago. He used an ingenious device. Rats were studied in pairs—an experimental rat and a control rat—each housed in a cage, one on each side of a flat circular plastic disk divided in half and suspended over water. Both rats had free access to their own supply of food and water, and both had been surgically implanted so that their sleep could be continuously monitored. The disk they lived on remained stable until the brain waves of the experimental rat showed the first signs of sleep. That automatically triggered the disk to begin to rotate slowly. Both rats, then, had to walk backwards or the motion of the platform would carry them forward and push them off into the water. This design was very successful in sleep depriving the experimental rat, whose sleep initiated the rotation of the disk. In spite of unlimited access to food and water, the experimental rats lost weight progressively and showed other signs of physical deterioration. They lost patches of fur, developed sores on their tails and paws and became much meaner and harder to handle. The control rat also had to walk or get a dunking, but since it was the experimental rat's attempt to sleep that set the platform into motion, the control rats got some sleep and survived. The experimental rats died within 3 weeks. What was the cause of death? Apparently, it was the failure of their body temperature to drop, which usually happens during sleep. No sleep equals no drop in temperature. Rats must sleep or die.

Humans also experience a drop in body temperature as we fall asleep, and it does not rise again until shortly before we wake up in the morning. This sleep-related decrease in temperature is more pronounced in those who describe themselves as good sleepers than it is in poor sleepers. When tested in the lab wearing rectal temperature probes (they were well paid), poor sleepers had higher core temperatures than did good sleepers and their all-night temperature charts showed flatter curves. Many of our mothers told us to open our bedroom windows at night—"Fresh air will make you sleep better." This certainly makes for chillier bedrooms, but our body temperatures do not follow the room temperatures closely. The reduction of the core body temperature relates to good sleep, not ambient temperature. Autopsies of the rats from Rechtschaffen's study indicated a failure to down-regulate internal temperature, which resulted in them running too hot for too long. They had a metabolic burn-out.

The news that rats died without sleep was impressive. Most interesting to me at the time was the finding that the rats' emotional behavior changed. As sleep deprivation accumulated, the experimental rats became so nasty and aggressive that they would bite right through the tough leather gloves lab assistants wore for their protection. But maybe rats when stressed get meaner just because they are rats. How about humans?

Health Problems Related to Short Sleep

What do we know about the effects of sleep loss on humans? There have been many studies of what happens when the number of sleep hours is reduced. Some of these were part of large-scale health surveys; others were small laboratory studies. One of the survey types, now a controversial classic, was conducted by the American Cancer Society on over a million people. The purpose was to find predictors of a later diagnosis of cancer by following a large, healthy sample over a 10-year period. Interviewers screened each participant to rule out those with a major health problem, including cancer, or who were taking medicine to control some diagnosed medical condition. There was only one exception; medication to control hypertension was permitted.

The survey asked only one question about sleep: "How many hours a night do you typically sleep?" Ten years later, when the interviewers contacted the original participants to conduct a follow-up survey, they found that those who had reported sleeping 6 hours or less had a higher mortality rate than expected for their age. However, they also found a higher death rate for those who slept more than 9 hours per night. This U-shaped curve, with higher mortality rates for both extremely short and long sleepers, has been found over and over, especially in men. If sleep is good for us, why is long sleep bad for us? We seem to need a balance between wake and sleep hours at a ratio of about 2:1.

What can studies of sleep deprivation in humans tell us about why a full night's sleep is so important? Some of the earliest of these studies, when REM was first discovered, were aimed at discovering why we seemed to need so much "dream time." These experiments targeted REM sleep preventing it by awakening the sleeper for 3 to 5 minutes, while not interfering with NREM sleep. Would that cause waking episodes of hallucinations? If REM and dreams help keep us in good mental health, would depriving sleepers of REM give us an experimental model of psychosis? The short answer is no. The most reliable effect of having less REM sleep, or less sleep of any kind, is "sleepiness," and that accounts for some of the behavioral effects we all notice after a bad night. Our minds drift off from whatever we are doing, especially during boring tasks. As our attention wanders, we make dumb mistakes and become irritated at having to correct these. But this is no help in understanding the contributions of a balance of hours asleep to hours awake in overall healthful functioning. Let's pick up some more clues from current research.

In a recent experiment by Karine Spiegel, of the University of Lyon in France, 11 young men, all of whom had passed a medical screening that pronounced them to be healthy, were allowed only 4 hours of sleep for 6 consecutive nights. At the end of the study, when they were screened again, a problem showed up. Their blood samples showed impaired glucose tolerance, a warning sign for the development of diabetes. This result was remarkable considering it happened after only a relatively short period of partial sleep loss. The good news was that this effect was completely reversible when these volunteers were allowed to resume sleeping without restriction.

It is considered unethical these days to extend sleep deprivation in research studies on humans just to see what happens. Researchers must submit their proposals to a committee charged with protecting volunteers from abuse.

These institutional research boards (IRBs) keep a watchful eye on researchers in order to assure the protection of human participants. Fortunately, we do not need to deprive people in a lab to study the effects of sleep deprivation because so many people do it voluntarily themselves. We can study them. When we consider the strong effect Spiegel found from a short period of partial sleep loss in the 11 healthy men alongside evidence from large community-based surveys asking about sleep habits and health, it becomes clear that there is a link between sleeping 5 hours or less per night and the onset of full-blown diabetes. Short sleepers polled in the Sleep Heart Health Study (implemented by the National Heart, Lung and Blood Institute) were 2.5 times more likely to be diabetic than those sleeping 7–8 hours nightly. This puts impaired glucose tolerance and diabetes close to the top of the list of known health problems that are clearly related to inadequate sleep.

Number 1 on that list is obesity. Here the dramatic finding of one study was that by age 27, those who sleep less than 6 hours a night are 7.5 *times more likely* to have a higher-than-healthy body mass index (BMI). An even larger study of over a thousand adults, whose sleep was recorded in their homes, found the fewest overweight people were those sleeping 7.7 hours—in other words, most overweight people did not get enough sleep. Which was cause and which effect?

The connection between short sleep hours and obesity has to do with the effect of sleep loss on hormones that control appetite (leptin suppresses appetite and ghrelin stimulates it). Short sleep led to increased appetite, and that was related to lower levels of leptin in short sleepers. This is part of an emerging picture of the causes of obesity—of course more factors are being studied every day. But the low leptin induced by sleep restriction has been confirmed by further studies. The Institute of Medicine's recent book *Sleep Disorders and Sleep Deprivation* sums up this work with the prediction that obesity will grow as we reduce our average hours of sleep; both of these troubling trends need our attention. We could say that short sleep equals a hungry wake-up. If you awaken hungry after a short night and have a coffee and doughnut breakfast, you can expect it will both put on pounds and put you at risk for diabetes.

Increased appetite following the selective loss of REM sleep was actually noted some 50 years ago in the very first laboratory study of "dream deprivation." Bill Dement published this finding in 1960. After just 3 to 5 nights of being awakened at each first sign that REM was about to begin, volunteers reported that they had increased appetites the next day, and showed a small weight gain at the end of the study, which took less than a week. They also reported experiencing increased anxiety. As mentioned, the increase in appetite has since been replicated, but the importance of the anxiety finding was not appreciated at the time. Dement himself noted the appetite increase and wondered whether feeding his volunteers when he woke them up to suppress REM would be a substitute for the missing dream time. If the volunteers ate instead of having REM and then did not experience the usual increase in REM sleep when they were allowed to sleep again without interruption, his hunch would be supported.

Dement tells the story of what happened in a charming book called *Some Must Watch While Some Must Sleep*. He consulted with a colleague, Dr. Charles Fisher, who agreed that they should give this food-for-REM-replacement a try. Dement then asked the next volunteer applying to take part in a study: "What is your favorite food?" "Banana cream pie," was the answer. Mrs. Fisher baked the pie. When the sleeper showed signs he was about to enter a period of REM sleep, he was awakened and asked the standard question: "What was going on in your mind just before I called you?" The first time, all went according to plan. The volunteer reported a little dream fragment, "I was walking down a street in Greenwich Village," and he was delighted to be offered a piece of pie to eat before going back to sleep. The same routine was repeated at each of the sleeper's attempts to achieve REM throughout the night. These attempts escalated during REM deprivation, and the time between REM periods shortened. Each time the sleeper was awakened, he could recall only a short snippet of a dream and gladly accepted another piece of pie. By the fourth awakening, the sleeper reported "I was having a cup of coffee and a cigarette." He ate the pie with less enthusiasm and commented, "I always have coffee and a cigarette at the *end* of meals [italics in the original]." The fifth time his dream report was more explicit: "I was given some spaghetti but was scraping it off the plate into a garbage can." He ate the fifth piece of pie reluctantly, leaving the crust. At the sixth awakening, he surprised the experimenter by saying: "Dr. Dement, I dreamed I was feeding *you* banana cream pie." Apparently he had had enough. Take note of the change—the subject displayed a marked shift in attitude. Like the rats, this sleeper showed signs of getting "fed up." The bad mood that follows interrupted sleep suggests that perhaps normal dreaming has a calming effect on emotion. Loss of REM may equal direct expression of negative mood. Remember that in Chapter 1, I noted that Snyder's healthy sleepers had more negative dream emotion than positive, at a 2:1 ratio. These findings offer another piece of evidence about what the mind is doing at night—regulating negative feelings, provided we get enough sleep.

All of the research evidence on the effects of short sleep on health was recently brought together by a distinguished group of scientists and published by the Institute of Medicine in the 2006 book, mentioned earlier, *Sleep Disorders and Sleep Deprivation: An Unmet Public Health Problem*. The book makes a compelling case that reduction of sleep hours is an important public health issue, and that sleep deprivation is at least partially responsible for the rise in some of our most troublesome health problems. As noted, there are strong links between short sleep and several of our most prevalent health problems: obesity, diabetes, hypertension, heart attacks, stroke, anxiety, and depressive mood. Some of these are primarily physical/medical problems, although behavior certainly contributes to them, whereas others are psychological/emotional problems. I will not review all of the evidence that documents the toll that short sleep takes on our physical health; instead, I will concentrate on how reduced amounts of sleep and the poor quality of the sleep hours we do get relates to waking changes in mood, impulsivity, self-esteem, and social relationships, all of which have been late in getting the research attention they deserve.

Look back at the diagram of a normal night of sleep in Chapter 1 (Fig. 1.2). It is clear that short sleep inevitably results in a reduction of the amount of REM, since most REM comes at the end of the night. If we go to bed later than usual but have to wake up at the usual time, REM sleep is sacrificed. If we go to bed at our regular time but have to wake an hour or two earlier to catch a plane or to make an early appointment, again our normal quota of REM will be reduced. If all is well, and these shifts in schedule are temporary, we can catch up the next night and get back on track. It is when we cannot get enough sleep night after night that we are at risk of disrupting the physical and emotional functions carried out in sleep, and most specifically in REM. We humans are a day–night system, with sleep and waking experiences interacting continuously. Our understanding of this is now rapidly increasing.

When Short Sleep Is Insomnia

Given that all people sleep badly some of the time, and some people sleep badly all of the time, we turn next to those who used to sleep well but who now sleep fewer than 6 or 7 hours despite trying desperately to get more sleep. (Of course, trying too hard is exactly the wrong way to encourage sleep. If we get angry about not being able to sleep it is better to get up and calm down before trying again.) Who is vulnerable to a diagnosis of so-called insomnia? What does this problem look like during a night in a sleep laboratory? What are the effects of reduced quality and quantity of sleep on how and what we dream? And finally, how does this, in turn, affect the next day's mood, attention span, learning ability, judgment, and general psychological functioning?

We will now take a turn through some of the short-term lab studies, along with others that stretch out over time in order to view the long-term psychological consequences of inadequate sleep. Since a little sleep loss leaves us crankier and more anxious the next day, will chronic sleep loss lead to more serious mood problems? Will abnormalities show up in the sleep studies of the chronically sleep deprived, in their brain imaging studies, and in dream disturbances? Research in this area has been so focused on sleep that dreaming has been under-represented. Later, I will look into just what is, or are, the functions of dreaming, since that is what gets hit hardest when sleep is short.

Insomnia is the "common cold" of sleep medicine; so common that roughly 58% of people surveyed at any one time report difficulties getting to sleep initially, staying asleep throughout the night, or waking too early without the ability to get back to sleep. If this goes on for 2 or more weeks it is diagnosed as insomnia. Also like the common cold, this sleep problem is made up of a variety of different types. One of these, for instance, relates to its frequency. Is the insomnia episodic, or is it a chronic problem?

Overall, the complaint of insomnia is by far more common in women than in men. The reason (or reasons, as there are likely more than one) for this gender difference is not yet settled. Some argue that since women are more help-seeking than men for all disorders this alone can account for their higher insomnia rate; women's insomnia may not be truly higher than it is in men— they simply report it more frequently to their physicians.

There is no doubt that gender-related hormonal differences also contribute to a higher rate of insomnia among women. Women's monthly menstrual cycles have sleep-related symptoms, as do changes that accompany pregnancy. The first trimester is characterized by increased sleepiness. Later, this becomes disrupted sleep, to say nothing of the challenge of finding a comfortable position for sleep with a 15-pound sack belted around the middle. Then there are the hot flashes of menopause, which are very disruptive to solid sleep, and which may go on for years.

Another contributor to high insomnia rates in women may be their expected role behaviors. Typically, women wake to breast-feed infants at night, are more likely to respond to the child who cries out in the dark, and stay awake listening for the teenager to get in after a late date. Women are also more likely to have their sleep interrupted by the snoring of a bed partner, and are more often the primary caretaker of an elderly parent who may have come to share the home, some of whom wander about at night. These gender-related social role differences are now less sharply defined as marriages have become more egalitarian. Since both partners have equal claims on their need for sleep when both are in the work force, more men now fetch the infant to be nursed, rise to change a diaper, or respond to the child who has a nightmare. Insomnia rates are higher in both men and women who lose a partner through widowhood or separation than in those who are married or single. The rates are also higher in the unemployed, and those at the lowest income levels. It seems that those who are most disadvantaged or distressed in waking suffer sleep that is lighter and more easily interrupted.

In a large survey study carried out by the National Institute of Mental Health, almost 8,000 men and women in three communities were interviewed about their sleep and mental health; they were followed up on a year later. Daniel Ford and Douglas Kamerow, the authors, divided these interviewees into four groups: those who had no sleep complaints at either their first or second interview, those who had a sleep complaint only in the first interview, those who had a sleep complaint only when interviewed the second time, and those who complained at both times.

These groupings revealed interesting results. One was that 69% of those who complained of insomnia at the first interview were no longer reporting this trouble a year later. That means that most people get over this problem in a relatively short time. However, there was a strong finding that those who reported insomnia only at the second interview, or at both time points, had a much higher rate of major depression or an anxiety disorder at the time of the second interview. In other words, persistent insomnia appears to be a risk factor for psychiatric diagnosis.

This study challenged the sleep research community to take insomnia seriously, to develop new treatments that might prevent the development of these more serious problems. The response was dramatic. Two different groups got to work—pharmacologists at developing newer, safer sleeping pills, and psychologists at developing behavioral treatments. Given the American propensity for a "quick fix," it is to be expected that the pharmacological solution to sleep troubles has become the most popular, so psychologists worked to sharpen and shorten their behavioral treatments. The problem is that without a clear understanding of the underlying reason for the sleep disruptions, it may not always be appropriate to treat patients with a sleeping pill or with a behavioral approach. What is more, without a control group with which to compare the results of treatments, some of the success claimed by each of these methods may actually be due to the natural return to good sleep, which often happens on its own. As the Ford and Kamerow study showed, some insomnia is chronic and not likely to be corrected easily. Insomnia patients can become quite frustrating for sleep clinicians, who are often unsure how best to be helpful.

I remember very clearly my first insomnia patient. She was a tough one for me. She was 48 years old, a married housewife, and had one grown daughter. She had only worked a short time in a clerical job before marrying young. With her daughter now out on her own, my patient was an "empty nester" who felt useless and acted the part. She reversed the mother–daughter roles and developed a dependent relationship on her daughter. The daughter helped her mother choose make-up and clothes to look more attractive and up-to-date. The patient was reluctant to commit to regular treatment hours, claiming she did not have a car of her own and had never learned to drive. Her husband drove the family car to work early, so the daughter undertook to teach her mother to drive and helped her pick out a used car. She was then able to come to her appointments on her own, but was always a fearful, timid driver. Once she got home, she told me her anxiety was not relieved. I asked her why not, and she told me then that as she approached her driveway she would look up at her bedroom window and say to herself, "There is my torture chamber."

No wonder she could not sleep. This woman did not need a sleeping pill or a short behavioral program; she needed something to do during the day that would give her a sense of pride in herself and some purpose. This is what we settled on as her treatment goal. She decided to volunteer in the gift shop of a local hospital, which transformed her basic self-definition. No longer was she a useless person; now that she felt useful and that her days were no longer empty, her sleep improved. Although neither of us thought this a perfect solution, no longer was sleep a nightly torture. It would have been easy to prescribe a sleep aid and send this woman on her way, but what she needed was far more complex.

The first rule of patient care is diagnosis before treatment. The second: Keep it simple, stupid. This is known as the KISS rule. Given that, much of insomnia is self-correcting after a short period; when it is not, it requires a keen understanding of what may be sustaining the problem. To answer this, a night in the sleep laboratory is rarely the first step. The lab is a high-tech and expensive test and one which, as experience tells us, often yields a better than usual night of sleep for many insomniacs. Simply removing these patients from the environment in which they now anticipate nothing but bad nights (like my patient who could not sleep in her "torture chamber") and placing them in a different place with an expert sleep technician standing by to watch over them all night, changes their expectations. Often patients relax in the lab and have their best night of sleep in years. In fact, when sleep techs ask the next morning "How was your night?" many an insomnia patient will answer wistfully, "Wonderful. Can I move in?" This contrast between bad sleep at home and good sleep in the lab adds to the skepticism some clinicians have about the complaint of insomnia— that it does not represent a "real" medical disorder. The paradoxical good lab sleep experienced by some of these patients underlines the need to conduct sleep studies in the home environment, but this option is resisted strongly by some professionals who argue that home studies are not sufficiently quality controlled. This despite the fact that one of the largest, multisite, federally funded research studies of sleep apnea (a breathing disorder of sleep) was carried out with only home-based equipment. There will be more opportunities for home-based studies of sleep patients when insurance companies allow coverage of these services.

In addition to uncharacteristically good sleep, another anomaly surfaces when insomnia patients are recorded in the laboratory to document their sleep difficulty. Some patients, who told us at their intake interview that they were unable to sleep at all, did sleep in the laboratory but later denied this. They had a real difference in perception from what we professionals call sleep and what they experienced. I learned this from an elderly, cranky patient who taught me a lesson. He was brought in to the Sleep Disorder Service by his son, with whom he lived. Both of them claimed that he did not sleep at all most nights. I booked him for a study and reviewed his sleep test the next morning before he left the lab. It showed his sleep was mostly light NREM (Stage 2) with some REM, but no deep sleep (slow-wave sleep; SWS). The patient refused to believe my verbal report. He adamantly insisted he was awake all night. It was a case of dueling definitions. I then showed him his recording and identified for him, with his son looking on, the sleep spindles and K complexes that indicate to sleep scientists that the brain is in Stage 2 sleep. He countered with his own evidence, saying he had heard my technicians phoning in their order for pizza to be delivered at 2 A.M. We were both right.

The explanation for this difference in what constitutes sleep may well be that, as we age, we lose the high-amplitude delta waves that define SWS. Although in some cases these waves are still slower than those of Stage 2 sleep, they are no longer high in amplitude, and it is this SWS that gives us the delicious sense of having been deeply unconscious. Men experience reduction of their delta sleep sooner than women, beginning in their early 40s. Light sleepers typically hover between wakefulness, Stage 1 and Stage 2, all night, and feel that this is not the sleep they remember from the good old nights of their youth. They actually are able to monitor off and on what is going on in the outside world; no wonder they feel, like my cranky patient, that they have not slept at all. Attempts to deepen the sleep of the elderly are an ongoing challenge, and many routes have been taken. In one, human growth hormone, which has a big outflow in SWS, was injected into elderly sleep volunteers to see if it would restore some deep sleep. It did not work.

What does work for some, and at least does no harm, is ensuring that the poor sleeper gets outdoors during the day for some exposure to the sun's bright light. Too many elderly (and in fact many of the rest of us) who are poor sleepers stay indoors, working or perhaps watching TV under dimly lit conditions. Sunlight helps differentiate day from night, regulating sleep–wake cycles. It also suppresses melatonin, a substance released as we doze off. Getting elderly people to walk or sit in the sun helps to keep them awake all day, and this, along with shortening their bedtime hours, builds up the pressure for more consolidated and deeper sleep. For some, I add the recommendation that they take a very hot bath 2 hours before bedtime. This should be a long soak of at least 20 minutes. This relaxes tense muscles and drives the core body temperature up by a degree or two. They are then instructed to do something relaxing for an hour and a half before going to bed. During that interval, their internal thermostat will have begun to regulate the too-high core temperature downward, dropping it lower than the base temperature. Then they will begin to feel sleepy and ready to fall asleep. This routine counteracts the too-high core temperature of the poor sleeper, which stays elevated all night, and keeping up the hot bath routine for about 2 weeks helps to reset the temperature cycle to drop as we fall asleep. What is more, it changes the mindset from an expectation of failure to a more positive disposition. The former insomniac is now a normal sleeper who looks forward to a good night's sleep.

Although a sleep laboratory test may become necessary if a short course of behavioral treatment is not effective, the first step in the diagnosis of insomnia is usually a more prosaic data gathering technique, a paper and pencil sleep log that the patient fills out at home each morning for 2 weeks. This gives the clinician some clues about what may be causing the problem and how to approach it. It is important to understand what happens when patients try to sleep in their own environments, the places where they must learn how to sleep more successfully. The log asks them to first note events of the day (did something unusual happen?), then what time they turned off the light for sleep; this indicates whether there is a regular bedtime at which the body has been trained to expect sleep. Next the log asks how much time passed before sleep occurred, how often they were aware of waking up during the night, how long it took for them to get back to sleep, what time they got out of bed to start the day, and how they felt in the morning. All these answers help to match the treatment to the problem. Is this a sleep-onset problem only? Or the opposite: Is it the end of the night that comes too soon? Is there a difference between the patients' sleep during the week and their weekend nights? Does the log show multiple awakenings, or what is known as "fragmented sleep"? And of course there are those with all of these complaints—trouble initiating sleep, staying asleep, waking too early, feeling like the dickens all day, and then dreading another night, which sure makes it hard to fall asleep. A vicious cycle has been set in motion.

Good programs have been developed to manage these problems, and many can be carried out on one's own. Numerous books outline the steps of these programs. However, chronic insomnia is sometimes resistant to treatment, and can seriously impact cognitive and emotional functioning during waking. Perhaps the most dramatic effect, as identified by the Ford and Kamerow study as an outcome of long-lasting inadequate sleep, is a diagnosis of major depression. This is the next step of our exploration into the contribution of sleep to understanding ourselves.

Sleep and Dreams in Depression | 4

He's simply got the instinct for being unhappy highly developed.

—Saki, *The Match-Maker*

Difficulty sleeping is a primary symptom of depression. In fact, this symptom is so common that it is often ignored, or it may cause sleep clinicians to pursue a diagnosis of some other disorder, one somewhat easier to treat. Is the poor sleep due to periodic limb movements of sleep (PLMS)? Maybe this is a breathing disorder, like sleep apnea? If it turns out that these are false leads, depression may be considered next. Not only does sleep become troubled long before the characteristic lack of interest in food, sex, social activity, and other symptoms become apparent; it is also the longest-lasting complaint of the depressed, often trailing on long after the patient's mood has improved and other hallmarks of the disorder are gone. Depression is for many a recurring disorder, and the insomnia of depression also waxes and wanes. When those who have had a depressive episode are functioning well they sleep better, but sleep worsens prior to the appearance of another episode. This predictive power of sleep difficulties was documented by Michael Perlis in a 1997 study of formerly depressed patients who were surveyed after they had completed Interpersonal

Psychotherapy (IPT) and had been in full remission for at least 4 weeks. Half of the sample had another episode of depression. They showed an increasing level of sleep disturbance over the 5 weeks preceding the onset of the new depression episode. The other half showed no sleep disturbance and did not suffer a recurrence. Neither group was on antidepressant medication or in psychotherapy during the follow-up period.

The most identifiable symptom of depression is the one that gives the name to the game. After all, this is a mood disorder. It begins with subtle indications: more crankiness and irritability before the sad, hopeless mood takes over. Once the black cloud descends, there follows a loss of interest in activities that had been sources of pleasure, decreased energy, a pervasive feeling of "tiredness," a poor appetite with weight loss, lessened or no interest in sex, withdrawal from social interactions, an unreasonable feeling of guilt or worthlessness, an impaired ability to concentrate and make decisions, and perhaps thoughts of or even plans and attempts to commit suicide. Could the persistent loss of good sleep be an underlying cause of this whole cascade of symptoms, affecting how we think, feel, define ourselves, and relate to others? We have had hints of this in some of the studies of short sleep; Rectschaffen's rats for instance (see Chapter 3). Now we turn to the sleep lab to look more closely at what ails the sleep and dreams of those suffering from clinical depression.

Sleep Studies of Depression

When patients complain of persistent poor sleep and report the waking symptoms of blue mood, loss of appetite, and so on, and a sleep study is ordered to help clarify the diagnosis, the recordings are likely to show two signs that mark the sleep as characteristic of major depression. These depression indicators were established first in severely depressed patients who were often hospitalized because they were judged to be suicide risks. In fact, the inpatient unit of the psychiatry service of the University of Pittsburgh had all their beds wired to record depressed patients' sleep every night during their stay. This yielded a lot of data that became the basis for a series of publications identifying those sleep characteristics specific to serious clinical depression. The first of these is the timing of the initial rapid eye movement (REM) episode of the night, which often starts too soon. These patients shift from light non-REM (NREM) sleep, Stage 1, and then to Stage 2, then straight into REM—without reaching Stages 3 and 4, slow-wave sleep (SWS). Their brain waves speed up, and heart rates and respiration become faster and more variable; a sudden loss of muscle tone is followed by flashing rapid movements of the eyes. REM is beginning, but less than 65 minutes after these patients fall asleep—not at the typical 90 minutes.

The more severe the depression, the earlier the first REM begins. Sometimes it starts as early as 45 minutes into sleep. That means these sleepers' first cycle of NREM sleep amounts to about half the usual length of time. This early REM displaces the initial deep sleep, which is not fully recovered later in the night. This displacement of the first deep sleep is accompanied by an absence of the usual large outflow of growth hormone. The timing of the greatest release of human growth hormone (HGH) is in the first deep sleep cycle. The depressed have very little SWS and no big pulse of HGH; and in addition to growth, HGH is related to physical repair. If we do not get enough deep sleep, our bodies take longer to heal and grow. The absence of the large spurt of HGH during the first deep sleep continues in many depressed patients even when they are no longer depressed (in remission).

The first REM sleep period not only begins too early in the night in people who are clinically depressed, it is also often abnormally long. Instead of the usual 10 minutes or so, this REM may last twice that. The eye movements too are abnormal—either too sparse or too dense. In fact, they are sometimes so frequent that they are called *eye movement storms*. To me they look like fireworks going off. What is going on then in their minds?

Waking these patients 5 minutes into the first REM sleep episode and asking what they are experiencing is disappointing. They typically have nothing to tell us. When depression is severe, this goes on throughout the night. This lack of dream recall in depression is important and has been found in study after study. Is it a reluctance to talk, to interact with the sleep researchers? Or, are these patients really not forming and experiencing any dreams?

Brain imaging technology has helped to shed light on this mystery. Scanning depressed patients while they sleep has shown that the emotion areas of the brain, the limbic and paralimbic systems, are activated at a higher level in REM than when these patients are awake. High activity in these areas is also common in REM sleep in nondepressed sleepers, but the depressed have even higher activity in these areas than do healthy control subjects. This might be expected—after all, these are people with a disorder of emotion. Another unexpected finding was that while in REM these individuals also show higher activity in the executive cortex areas, those associated with rational thought and decision making. Nondepressed controls do not exhibit this activity in their REM brain imaging studies. This finding has been tentatively interpreted by Eric Nofzinger, another of the University of Pittsburgh team who has done much depression research, as perhaps a response to the excessive activity in the areas responsible for emotions.

This high level of activity in the cognitive control brain areas may be what blocks the development of dream scenarios and the subsequent emotional expression that usually takes place during REM. Luckily for those researchers interested in dreaming, when the depression is not very severe (when the symptoms are present but not disabling), we are able to collect reports of depressed peoples' dreams to study how their minds are working in REM. We then can compare these to dreams of control subjects who are not depressed. We have followed groups who are symptomatic of depression but still functional enough to remain living at home and to hold a job. Studying this population of people has helped fill in our understanding of the mind asleep. We turn to them next.

Dreaming in Depression

For almost 30 years and with the support of federal funding, I did a series of studies on moderately depressed men and women who were not patients but volunteers paid to sleep in the lab and share their dreams. Fired by my persistent interest in tracing the interaction between the mind states across the 24 hours of the day, I wanted to see how a mood disorder that affects cognition, motivation, and most of all the emotional state during waking, shows itself in dreams. We know that the REM sleep of the depressed has abnormalities, but we have very little information about what is going on inside their sleeping minds. We also know from the earlier attempts of others to study this population that the dream recall of the depressed is poor. This was difficult research to do, as most of the medications that are prescribed to relieve depression also suppress REM sleep. However, some interesting early research on cats that were surgically REM-deprived showed that following recovery, the cats had a strong increase in appetite, sex drive, and motor activity. That suggested that the REM suppression effect of antidepressant drugs might be the mechanism responsible for reinvigorating depressed patients—at least in those who had a good response to their medications.

Gerald Vogel, a psychiatrist at Emory University, took this idea and, between 1975 and 1980, carried out the most exciting sleep research that had been done on depression until then. He found a way around the ethical problem of stopping depression medication for research purposes. His sleep lab was based in a psychiatric hospital where most new patients were either not yet on medicine or were routinely tapered off of it before switching to new drugs. Dr. Vogel could study patients while they were drug-free, and since they were in need of hospital care, they were also seriously depressed. If their REM sleep was abnormal, what would happen if Vogel deprived them of REM extensively? In Bill

Dement's study, normal volunteers had an increase in appetite after just 3 to 5 nights of REM deprivation. What if Dr. Vogel carried this out longer? It was understood that this was not a risky study; the patients were in a protective environment, and the loss of REM sleep by the awakening technique could be reversed with a rebound of increased REM sleep for a few nights once the participants were allowed to sleep naturally again. The one drawback was that, when REM is prevented, it takes more and more awakenings to keep people out of REM sleep. Vogel did not want this to be a sleep deprivation study; he wanted to test just the effects of REM loss on depressive symptoms. He solved this problem in a most ingenious way: He set a limit of no more than 30 awakenings per night and carried on the REM deprivation of the patients for 6 consecutive nights, allowing them the seventh night off, while still being recorded, but without interruption. This allowed for only a partial REM rebound, and Vogel was able to continue the deprivation procedure for 3 weeks—much longer than if he had continued REM deprivation without that seventh-inning break.

Being an experienced sleep researcher, Dr. Vogel designed this study to have a control group, a group of similar patients who received only NREM awakenings of equal number. Each group had 17 patients. After 3 weeks of REM deprivation, half of those in the experimental group were judged by the staff to be well enough to go home with no further treatment. None of the control group had symptom improvement. Those who did not respond to the experimental treatment were put next on one of the traditional therapies. The controls were then crossed over into the REM deprivation protocol. Again, half of the group responded with a reversal of their symptoms. They too passed the judgment of the staff as being ready for discharge and left the hospital. What were the differences between those that responded positively and those who did not? Dr. Vogel looked carefully at the data and found that the patients who improved were those who, when prevented from having early REM by the awakenings, built up pressure for more REM sleep at the end of the night (as is the case in normal sleepers). In other words, the good responders normalized their sleep on the seventh uninterrupted night. This effect took 3 weeks to achieve (6 nights of REM deprivation followed by a seventh of regular sleep, repeated three times), but most antidepressant medications take even longer to produce a therapeutic effect.

Perhaps Vogel's patients had only a temporary boost in mood, energy, and appetite, just to avoid having to be awakened 30 times per night. This is not so. These patients returned for follow-up visits and did as well as those who left the hospital after more conventional treatments. This all sounds very exciting, but these findings are difficult to explain. Not all antidepressant drugs that are successful in relieving depression are REM sleep suppressors, and not all depressed patients respond to the same treatment type. Furthermore, sustained REM deprivation is not an easy treatment to apply clinically. This study stands as a landmark, but it left a good deal of work to do in understanding major depressive illness. My disappointment was that the Vogel study did not address the psychological component: the night-life of the depressed.

I was eager to tackle that gap in our information about dreams during depression. This was particularly intriguing to me because we know that about 60% of those who have a depressive episode recover without any formal treatment. That figure was supported in a study of widows by another psychiatrist, Paula Clayton. I wanted to find a similar group who were depressed following a major life event but not taking any antidepressant medication. This time, the aim was to investigate the subjects' dreams over an extended period to find out if they had any helpful effect on emotional functioning. I wanted to use a real-life problem, one strongly associated with the onset of depression, rather than creating an artificial experimental situation to induce an emotional state in the lab. Many such experiments had previously failed to make any impact on dreams. People have a remarkably strong ability to ignore our attempts to influence what they dream about, and instead go right on dreaming those of their own making, centered on their personal concerns. That teaches us something humbling, and the best experimental dream studies have recognized this fact.

The event I chose to work with was divorce from a first marriage. There was a lot of that going on when I began these studies back in 1978. At that time, the divorce rate had reached 50%, and the rate of depression in those with bad marriages was 25 times higher than in those with good marriages. Divorce, an event closely related to the onset of a depressive episode, had several advantages for a naturalistic study. Recovery from depression takes time, about 6 months to a year, whether in response to an antidepressant, to psychotherapy, or to unknown and perhaps naturalistic factors. This gives us time to watch changes in dreams take place. Like the death of a spouse, we know that not all people "get over" a depression associated with loss of a loving relationship on their own. Who does, and who does not, and what role REM sleep and dreaming play in this process were the questions I wanted to answer. I continued these studies up until 2005, by which time it had become harder to recruit divorcing volunteers. (Too many of those breaking-up had never been legally married.)

Those who took part in my studies were not patients but members of the community, who responded to a newspaper advertisement. The ad asked for volunteers who were feeling blue over a separation or divorce and who were willing to spend nights in a sleep lab for a project concerned with their sleep and dreams. They would be paid for their time. Many who responded were clinically depressed, although they did not recognize that their sadness was beyond that which would be expected following a failed relationship. All were questioned by a member of our team trained to administer the standard interview used to diagnose psychiatric disorders (the Structured Clinical Interview for DSM Disorders or SCID). Some volunteers did not meet the criteria for depression, and they became our divorcing control group. None had been treated either with drugs or psychotherapy, and they were not seeking treatment. I made it clear that this was not what I offered. This was ideal for my purposes; I wanted to study whether there is a natural healing process that could be detected in dreams.

Those who we selected were ordinary men and women going through one of life's most difficult legal and emotional processes. Some had initiated the breakup, while others were the ones who had been left behind. All were attempting to adjust to their new circumstances. Divorce often means a loss of a home, as well as loss of a partner. Most were working, trying to get their lawyers' attention, organizing finances so they could pay their bills. Those with kids had the added burden of single parenthood and working out visitation schedules. Almost all shed tears as we discussed the history of the marriage during our first interview. Clearly, they were deeply affected by the stress of this unhappy ending to the dream of "for ever after."

What motivated these volunteers to come in and to keep coming back for the length of the study? For some, it was the money, as many were hard up. Most mentioned it was their trouble sleeping and the opportunity to talk about the marriage failure with an understanding but nonjudgmental person that interested them. They hoped that since this was a "sleep study" it would yield useful information for us and for them.

Working Through Divorce in Dreams

Despite differences in terminology, all the contemporary theories of dreaming have a common thread—they all emphasize that dreams are not about prosaic themes, not about reading, writing, and arithmetic, but about emotion, or what psychologists refer to as *affect*. What is carried forward from waking hours into sleep are recent experiences that have an emotional component, often those that were negative in tone but not noticed at the time or not fully resolved. One proposed purpose of dreaming, of what dreaming accomplishes (known as the mood regulatory function of dreams theory) is that dreaming modulates disturbances in emotion, regulating those that are troublesome. My research, as well as that of other investigators in this country and abroad, supports this theory. Studies show that negative mood is down-regulated overnight. How this is accomplished has had less attention.

I propose that when some disturbing waking experience is reactivated in sleep and carried forward into REM, where it is matched by similarity in feeling to earlier memories, a network of older associations is stimulated and is displayed as a sequence of compound images that we experience as dreams. This melding of new and old memory fragments modifies the network of emotional self-defining memories, and thus updates the organizational picture we hold of "who I am and what is good for me and what is not." In this way, dreaming diffuses the emotional charge of the event and so prepares the sleeper to wake ready to see things in a more positive light, to make a fresh start. This does not always happen over a single night; sometimes a big reorganization of the emotional perspective of our self-concept must be made—from wife to widow or married to single, say, and this may take many nights. We must look for dream changes within the night and over time across nights to detect whether a productive change is under way. In very broad strokes, this is the definition of the mood-regulatory function of dreaming, one basic to the new model of the twenty-four hour mind I am proposing. Now on to the first study.

Study 1: Dreams of Depressed and Nondepressed Divorcing Volunteers

The first question to be answered in this test was, will this strategy work? Will waking *moderately* depressed sleepers from their REM sleep yield enough dream reports to test whether they dream differently from those experiencing the same event (in this case divorce) without depression? Are there differences in what they dream? Do they, for example, dream more often of their departing partners? Is the expression of emotion in the dream an important aspect of recovery from an episode of depression? What kinds of dreams have a positive effect on mood in the short term (the next morning) and in the long run (to help resolve the depression)? My hypothesis was that those whose waking psychological state was moderately depressed would give us a window into how sleep and dreams reflect a major disruptive life change, and eventually help reshape the organization of the self to, in effect, get over a depression.

Research is often a messy, trial-and-error business. At least for me, I learn as I go, and often what I learn is how I should have designed a study in the first place. That was true of the first stab I made at exploring what was going on in the minds of these people during their REM sleep. Of the 60 who started in the first study, 23 women and 26 men completed it. They slept in the laboratory for 3 nights at the beginning of their divorce process and returned a year later for their final 3 nights and another diagnostic evaluation. Thirty-one of the participants were diagnosed as depressed initially, and 18 were not depressed at the start of the study. One year later, 11 of the original 31 were still depressed, but the remaining 20 had recovered. That gave us a basis for comparing the dream differences between these two groups, with an emphasis on the emotions expressed in dreams, whether they dreamed of their marriage partners, and how that related to whether they recovered.

Two research assistants, who did not know the depression status of the dreamers, rated the dream transcripts. They scored each dream for the intensity of the emotion—none, moderate, or strong—and whether the ex-spouse was a character in the narrative. The dreamers also rated their own dreams at the time they answered the call on the intercom. Once they completed telling all they could remember, they were asked, "Would you say that dream was positive (pleasant), neutral, or negative (unpleasant)?" and "Would you say that dream was highly emotional, mildly emotional, or not at all emotional?" There were big differences between the dreams of the 31 depressed and those of the 18 healthy controls. At the start of the study, 39% of dreams were rated as unpleasant by the depressed volunteers, but just 14% were rated as unpleasant in the healthy controls. Both groups were going through a divorce, but waking mood colored the dreams of the depressed in darker hues. Half of the depressed group dreamed of their ex-spouses and half did not. These two subgroups began the study as equally depressed on two standard tests used to assess depression (the Beck Depression Inventory and the Hamilton rating scale). But those whose ex-partner did appear in their dream reports experienced stronger emotions in their dreams, and more of them were *no longer* depressed at the close of the study. Furthermore, in their last interview, members of this group were judged to be making better progress adjusting in their waking lives—coping better at work, with their finances, with their children, and even dating. What was the nature of these dreams of their former spouses? Here are two from those who were initially depressed but later recovered.

> I had to tell my boyfriend I couldn't see him because work
> has to take priority because of the financial mess my
> husband left me in. I was upset and thought, "You bastard,
> you got in the way again."

> I was having a fight with my husband; yelling and angry.
> He's not taking good care of himself, overworking. He was
> running to me not feeling well, started collapsing. I was on
> the phone trying to make a call. I sat him down on a pile of
> something. I was persuading him to stay put while I called a

cab to take him to the hospital. I was holding him up and I
said, "I have to go back and close the door."

The dreams of both of these volunteers expressed anger at their ex-spouse,
and in them the dreamers appeared to be actively trying to move on with their
lives; they were still bothered by a lack of closure to the marriage.

Now take a look at two dreams reported by healthy (nondepressed) controls
featuring the ex-spouse. Note the difference.

I was invited to dinner by a friend and she said "Sorry, so
and so (name of my ex) is not coming, so no dinner." So I
went home to bake a cake for myself.

[I was] taking a Christmas tree in my car to throw it out.
I was in the truck my wife and I owned, and the fender got
bent. I was complaining that you have to pay so much for
things, and they don't hold up right. It felt like tinfoil.

No anger is expressed here. Although both dreamers seem to recognize the
negative consequences of being divorced, losing out on social events and paying
a high price for things that do not last, they calmly take action to take care of
themselves.

The study results looked promising. We could collect dreams from depressed
individuals that reflected their present emotional state, and I was eager to get
on with testing whether dreams contributed to the regulation of negative mood.
It took 5 years for me to get this far. It was 1983, but I felt I needed to step back
and take a look at how dreams relate to waking mood when we are *not* going
through a major change in our lives. In other words, I needed a baseline study
of some well-functioning sleepers, along with more information about what
was on their minds right before sleep—specifically, how they were feeling and
whether their current feelings related to their dreams.

Study 2. Dreams of Healthy Volunteers and Their Mood Before and After Sleep

This time I invited sixty healthy adults, 30 men and 30 women, to spend just
2 nights sleeping in the lab. All were high-functioning young adults enrolled in
a professional graduate education program. We screened them to make sure
they had no history of depression and were in good mental and physical health.

Since even the best of us can have an unexpected bad day, meet some bump in the road, get in a fender bender, hear bad news, and still be upset come nightfall, we used two tests to measure their states of mind before sleep. The first was a measure of their current concerns (CC), a test I designed to tap into those issues that were on their minds each night, and how strongly they felt about each one. There were 12 items in all, on issues such as health, finances, friends, love life, and more. The volunteers were asked to rate their current degree of concern on a 5-point scale ranging from 1 (not at all concerned) to 5 (extremely concerned). The other test was a well-known test of moods, the Profile of Mood States (POMS), used to evaluate the present degree of volunteers' moods, both good and bad, including depression. They took this test again in the morning. These two instruments would give us a better understanding of what the sleepers' main concerns were at the time, on what topic and to what degree, what emotion they were experiencing before sleep, and whether the emotions were more muted next morning. I wanted to know if the issues that concerned the volunteers most strongly would transfer into sleep and influence their dreams. And if it did, would their mood change for the better the following day?

The first night, the volunteers slept without any interruption to get used to wearing the monitors. On night 2 they were awakened during each REM period and asked to report what was on their minds. We followed the same dream collection routine that I had used with the divorcing sample in Study 1, asking them the same questions after each report: Was this a positive, neutral, or negative experience? Was it highly emotional, mildly emotional, or neutral? We found some interesting things that I had not predicted. (When this happens I have been known to exclaim with great enthusiasm, "Hey, hey! Cute data!" This got to be a lab joke. My assistants, Jenny and Julie, told me when they were asked what they did in the lab, they would answer "Oh, I look for cute data." These unanticipated "goodies" are the fun of research.)

Although none of the volunteers for this new study were in any crisis, the women scored higher on the depression scale of the POMS before sleep than did the men, although all of them were in the low range. This was not surprising, as women have a much higher rate of clinical depression than do men, and in general women are more self-critical. Nonetheless, in this healthy group, depression scores went down in both genders when they repeated the POMS test next morning. The same was true on the second night, the night we woke them for reports from each REM period. That night the women tested a little higher on depression than did the men, although both showed improved mood the next day. What was going on during the night that might account for this?

We split the group into two, those whose POMS tests showed no disturbing mood before sleep and those who had some elevated score, and examined their answers to our question about whether the dreams they reported were positive, negative, or neutral. Both groups had neutral dreams and dreams they could not remember in about equal numbers, so we concentrated on those they considered to be positive and negative. There was a big difference between the groups in the proportion of positive and negative dreams experienced during the first and last half of the night. Sure enough, the findings made sense (cute data!). Those who had no disturbed mood before sleep had predominantly more positive than negative dreams both in the first and second half of the night. Those who had some mood disturbance before sleep had dreams they rated as negative in the first half of the night, and positive dreams predominated in the second half of the night. What is more, overnight improvement in their waking mood scores was related to the emotional tone of their dreams in the second half of the night. *The higher the percent of positive dreams from the last two REM periods, the more improved the sleepers' morning moods.* This told us that within a healthy group with stable lives we could anticipate that waking mood improves from night to morning, and that this relates somehow to experiencing more positive dreams before waking up. Good news!

Let us go back for a moment to Study 1, to the sleepers who were not in a stable state, and were instead in the process of a major disruption in their lives— divorce. We performed the same analysis of emotional tone in the dreams these people had reported in the first and last half of the night, comparing these patterns to those reported in Study 2 by the well-functioning volunteers. We wondered if the pattern of the emotional tone of the dreams would predict who got over the depression and who did not. If the volunteers in Study 1 regulated their moods by shifting their dream stories from those with negative feelings at the beginning of the night to more positive dreams in the second half of the night, would they have a better chance of reorganizing their emotional memory system, and, over time, put the depression behind them?

Now we had three groups to compare: the controls who were divorcing but not depressed, those who were divorcing and depressed but recovered 1 year later, and those divorcing and depressed who showed no improvement in mood after 1 year. These groups showed interesting differences in their own ratings of the emotional tones of their dreams on the very first night of lab dream reporting. Again, we looked at the percentage of dreams that the dreamers called positive, negative, and neutral, and those they could not recall at all. We concentrated on the ratio of positives and negatives in the first half of the night and in the second half to test for any change in emotion, or lack of it, across the night. The healthy divorcing controls had more positive dream reports than negatives in the first half of the night, and these increased in the second half, from 12% to 19%. The depressed who would recover 12 months later had a pre-dominance of negative dreams in the first half of the night, but these reduced by half in their last two dream reports, from 19% to just 8%. Their positive dreams went up a little, from 9% to 13%. The negative dreams of those who were depressed and stayed depressed increased in proportion as the night went on. These doubled from 12% to 24% by the end of the night, with only a small improvement in the proportion of positive dreams from 12% to 15% (Fig. 4.1).

The results of the two studies were promising enough for me to ask for funding to take on a second study of men and women going through divorce. It was now 1994, and I had been at this for 16 years. It was slow work; we had only one bed devoted to research, as our lab was primarily for clinical diagnostic sleep studies of outpatients. But depression was, and still is, a major health problem, and I felt the work I was doing was unique. We had not used any mood scales in Study 1, and I believed it was important to get a closer look at the moods the subjects were in before sleep and how these change from night to morning. This time we would use both the POMS (mood) test and the CC (concerns) measure I had developed for the high-functioning volunteers, and which had before given us useful data. We added three new items to the list of

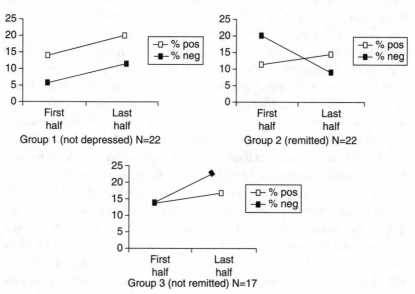

FIGURE 4.1 Percent of positive and negative dream affect by half-night in divorce volunteers

concerns, to tap into the degree of focus on the divorce: ex-spouse, lawyer, and loneliness. This way we could look at whether the level of concern on these more specific items dropped following dreams about the ex-spouse. I was also keen to find out whether embedding their concern about the ex-partner in a dream plot that included older memories contributed to diffusing the sleepers' negative mood, thereby helping to improve their morning mood and change their self-concepts over time. What can we learn about the process of moving from waking into sleep to dreaming, then to the morning after, by looking at the pattern of change over time when the sleeping mind improves waking mood—and when it does not? We have more cute data to share and more inside looks into the dream lives of those retooling their self-concept.

Over the years that I worked on the function of dreaming problem, I made changes in the design of this study on the basis of the results we were getting. For instance, I found that I did not need to follow volunteers for as long as a year to determine who would get better and who would not when no formal treatment was involved. Five months was enough. At that 5-month mark, 65% of those who had been depressed at the start in Study 1 no longer met the criteria for this diagnosis. That was the good news. The bad news was that when I applied for approval for my next study, my university's Institutional Review Board (IRB) gave me a very hard time. How could I justify not treating those I knew to be depressed, even if they themselves were unaware that they met this diagnosis and had not asked for help? It was a serious ethical concern. The board worried that if even one of my volunteers committed suicide, or just made a serious attempt, the hospital and I would likely be sued. They were not impressed that, out of the 130 divorcing people I had already studied, only two had voluntarily admitted themselves to the hospital for psychological reasons. Both were men whose mood improved after a short stay. They signed themselves out of the hospital within 48 hours, and continued on in our study. A psychiatrist on the research team checked up on all the volunteers routinely in person, and I was monitoring their sleep and dreams for signs of trouble.

The IRB members were still not willing to allow my research to go forward unless I provided treatment for those with a diagnosis of major depression. Fortunately, I reached a compromise that was acceptable. I added an item to the consent form volunteers signed stating that if they, or we the researchers, felt they needed some professional help during the course of the study, I would provide resources. Only a few took me up on that offer. Those who did asked for the name of a professional who could help their children, who were having adjustment problems. None asked for themselves. I did offer a few who were still in poor psychological shape at the end of the study the opportunity to work with me at no cost. I used their dream transcripts and focused on their unhappy dreams in order to help empower them to change their dreams for a more self-affirming result.

Now, on to Study 3. One of the most important tenets of research is replication. When a new finding is announced, scientists believe in remaining skeptical until that finding is confirmed in a second study. If the second study fails to report the same findings, either the original or second investigator may be wrong about his or her conclusions. Study 3 was our attempt to replicate our own findings on the role of dreaming in regulating negative emotion.

Study 3: Dreams of the Ex-spouse During Divorce

We have seen some cute data up to this point showing that high-functioning people with little ongoing negative mood before sleep (sadness, anger, anxiety) have mostly pleasant dreams and wake up in a good mood. Those with a mild amount of unresolved negative mood before sleep begin the night with negative dreams but end it with more positive dreams; they too wake up in a better mood than they were in the night before. Among those whose low mood qualifies as major depression, some do and some do not regulate negative dreams within the night; those who do not, wake without any improvement in the gloomy way they perceive the world and their place in it.

In our final study of divorcing volunteers, we screened and accepted 30 participants; 20 who were clinically depressed and 10 who were not. They all took the CC (current concerns) test each night and the POMS test both before and after sleep. They spent 2 nights in the lab at three time points: Month 1, Month 2, and Month 4. The first night, Night 1, was always a sleep-through night to allow the sleepers to acclimate themselves to sleeping in the lab. On Night 2, we woke them during each REM period to ask for a report. Having three sets of dreams gave us a closer look at how these dreams changed over time. In Study 1, we had collected dream reports at the beginning of the study and at the end, a full year later. This time the study lasted only 5 months, but we had three sets of dreams to examine. When we reassessed these volunteers at the end of the study, 12 who had been depressed were functioning well, but eight were still not over the depression. Would the subjects' first dream reports predict who would be in which state 5 months later?

The mood tests that the volunteers completed before and after each night revealed dramatic differences between those who would recover from their depression and those who would not. On the morning after their first sleep night at Month 1, all 20 of the depressed scored their mood as less depressed than the night before. When they came in the following night for the REM collections, the evening mood scores of those who went on to recover were the same as their morning scores; they had maintained their improved mood all day. After sleeping through the next night, their moods had improved further, as indicated by their morning POMS depression scale scores.

In the other group (the volunteers who would not recover from depression over the next 5 months), although their morning mood scores had improved after their first full night of sleep, they had lost that improvement by nightfall. When they came in for Night 2 they were as depressed as they had been before going to sleep on Night 1. Both groups (those who would recover and those who would not) continued the same pattern of changes in mood at Month 2 and Month 4. Those who were getting over the depression made progressive improvement over each night and maintained their gains during the day, and again those who would not recover did improve their mood with sleep, but failed to retain this progress during their wake time. They were as badly off before sleeping each night as they had been at the start of the study (Fig. 4.2). Was something important going on in between the night and morning tests of the improving group that was not occurring for the group that remained clinically depressed?

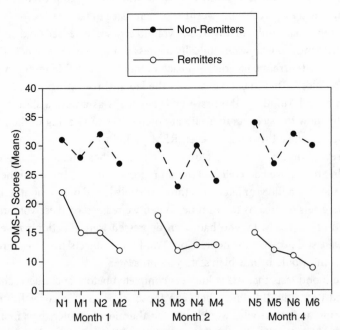

FIGURE 4.2 Overnight (night, morning) change in depressed mood in nonremitters and remitters

First, we looked at both groups before sleep responses to the current concerns questionnaire. Regardless of the items they picked as one or more of their current concerns, those who would not recover gave their concerns the highest rating—5, or extremely concerned. Did they dream about their former spouses? The 20 depressed volunteers split right down the middle—ten did and ten did not, at least on the nights when we collected their REM reports. Those who dreamed of the former partner had higher scores on the CC ex-spouse item than those who did not; their average concern score on the ex-spouse item was 4 at all three monthly testing points, in contrast those who had no dreams featuring ex-spouses were less concerned about them in waking. Their average score was 2.6 at Month 1, and went down to 1.8 on the last night at Month 4. Their level of concern about their exes when tested in waking times was strongly related to whether or not they dreamed of them.

Now let us look at the dreams themselves. What about them seemed to help these volunteers' recovery and what did not? Remember, we were not considering real-life issues such as payment of child support or giving each other a hard time—just how their degrees of concern and emotional states before sleep related to the images from memory that were displayed as a dream. We also wanted to know whether the dreams contributed to revisions in how they saw themselves, and consequently how they might handle difficulties in relationships in more positive ways in their waking lives.

Dreams of the Former Partner

Here are examples of dreams from two women who did not recover from their depression within 5 months (NR).

> NR1: I was dreaming about my husband who was dating this
> girl that he works with and him taking her out. That's all I
> can remember.
>
> Q: Anything else?
>
> NR1: He was just taking her out, meeting her at our house.
> I was just sitting in my house in my living room, and he was
> going out the door with this girl.

The husband leaves with a younger woman. The dreamer is passive and unemotional.

NR2: My kid's father got some shoes that we bought. He was just looking at shoes we bought for my sister. He brought them out while we were eating. I was sitting at the table eating.

The ex-spouse is identified only as the father of her children. They do not interact. The dreamer expresses no emotion. Both dreams are short, flat in feelings, and the dreamer is passive in action. Next are examples of dreams from two women who did recover from their depression (R).

R3: I was fleeing from something with my daughter and my son on a dark street in a suburban area, but in an Indian or Asian community with barbed wire around the fence. My son needed to use the bathroom and my daughter needed water for her dog. I knocked on the door of this house and an old woman answered, and I asked her for help, but a man came to the door and said "No." I asked him, "Why not?," and he said "You would have to be my wife." I didn't know what to do. Then we were backtracking through a field and shots were being fired all around. Then we were in a room where a dance was being planned. I was telling my ex-husband that I would only be staying for 5 minutes, and he said "Fine," like he didn't care. I knew that his new girlfriend would be there and they would be dancing. I felt resentful. I didn't want to see that.

The setting is from her past. She was raised in South Africa. The dreamer is active in trying to cope with the children's needs under what she perceives to be dangerous circumstances. When help is denied, she understands why she is now an outsider but continues on, finds the ex-spouse in a new relationship. She recognizes this and expresses her negative feelings of resentment.

R4: I was at the house I grew up in—and it was—there was a party for me, and it was almost like I had come home from a long time ago—I mean I haven't lived there since high school. But I went back to a party and a lot of people from high school I had known as a child had come back, so it was kind of like I was going to see all those people from when I was younger, from grade school, junior high school and, and then my ex-husband was there but I only saw him for a

minute and then I didn't really talk to him at all. I just saw
him for a minute and then he was gone. I know that's not
much but that's all I can remember, really. It's kind of weird
but this just came back. I have no idea where this fits in but
there was a woman who had on these weird looking shoes,
I remember that. They were pointy, and she had on a woven
hat that covered all her hair. She just had on some suede
brown shoes, pointy shoes, she had socks, really thick socks
on, with the shoes. Two men were trying to talk to her,
almost like they were trying to pick her up, and she
recognized that it wasn't a good situation, and she turned
around and disappeared into the crowd. It was more of a
street scene outside with a lot of people. It was almost like
I was watching a movie but I was glad she disappeared into
the crowd because I was not trusting the two men who were
trying to talk to her. The party was kind of good, to see
people I grew up with, that was good and then when I found
out that my ex-husband was there, I was kind of like I'll go
down and say hello to him, but once I saw him he did
something strange, so it was like, oh yah, whatever, so. He
exposed himself. I was embarrassed, but I wasn't you know
embarrassed for me, I was embarrassed for him. And it was
kind of like, well—I'm leaving now. I mean it bothered me
that he had done it, but it really wasn't any reflection on me.

This dream setting is also from an earlier time in the dreamer's life, and she
is happy before a second scene in which she expresses distrust of men's inten-
tions. The third scene returns to the first party where her ex-spouse is seen as
behaving inappropriately, justifying her distancing herself from him. She
expresses a range of emotions—happy at the party, glad the woman escaped,
embarrassed by her husband—and she is active in response to his behavior.

Differences between the dreams of the not recovered (NR) and the recovered (R) women are easy to spot. Those recovering experienced much longer,
more dramatic dreams, with complex plots and changes of scene. They include
many more characters. They both include images drawn from older memories
mixed with current issues. Both express how they feel about the ex-partner's
behavior.

The recovering women appeared to be working out their negative feelings
about the former spouse explicitly in their dream scenarios, and the first two
nonrecovering dreamers did not. They express neither emotion in their dreams

nor any complex blending of present images with past memories, as do the recovering women.

Here are two more examples of dreams featuring the former partner. This time the dreamers are healthy divorcing controls (C). The first is the dream of a woman; the second is a dream from a man. Neither was depressed at any of the three assessment points in the study. Let's see what is different about the way these nondepressed people dream about their former spouse.

> C5: This one is very vivid. I was at home and I had gone into my bedroom and my niece was playing in my closet and she had made a total mess. I told her she could play there as long as she cleaned up her mess. . . . Oh God, I remember my bedroom was a total mess, everything was everywhere. And I was showing her some lingerie I had bought, and then she told me she was going to get a boob job and we were talking about the doctor she was going to go to and he was going to charge a hundred thousand dollars. I was talking to my friend, and my niece was still in the closet playing with toys. How bizarre. A friend of mine who is a plastic surgeon somehow popped his head into the conversation, and was telling her that, you know, a hundred thousand dollars is too much to pay and that was not the standard price, the going price, and she was rationalizing it, saying the guy was really good. What a bizarre dream [laughing]. For some reason my ex was there, he was still in the house. I don't remember why. I had the door locked to my bedroom, which is where I was at. I didn't want him to see the lingerie I was showing my friend [uproarious laughter]. It was Valentine's Day lingerie, that cheap stuff, you know [giggling], trashy stuff. It obviously wasn't for him [laughing]. That was a pleasant dream.

This dreamer reports a complex dream with many characters and time references to past, present, and future. She expresses a range of emotions in response to how she copes with different problems. She is tolerant but firm with her niece, she is accepting of her friend's decision, and enjoys her power to exclude the ex-spouse from her future.

The next dream was reported by a man from the healthy control group. His ex-wife is a dream character.

C6: I was dreaming about a fight between my wife and another woman who I was dating. The woman had a name that was the same as the name of a woman I knew a long time ago, but she was not the same woman, she didn't look the same. I was at this woman's house, and we were becoming romantic and then the woman asked if we could stop until another time, and then not long after that I was on the phone. I don't know how all that came about to be on the phone with my wife, and then she called or not called but was on the phone with this other woman and they were arguing, right . . . and I got back on the phone, and my wife was belittling the other woman right when you woke me up. Before that, I had an extended dream about a premonition about what was going to happen in the future. I had a friend who met me at a bar for lunch and we were eating lunch at this crowded bar and he was ten minutes late in arriving and we were eating and we were talking about all kinds of things and we transitioned into knowing that someone was going to die and we knew where and what day and not how. It seemed I had just watched this movie and Clint Eastwood was in this movie and he knew someone was going to die in this movie and he went there to watch this happen and it was a flood that broke through the side of a ship. And water was starting to come in from a lot of directions and he stood there for a while. That happened right before I was with the woman. It jumped from water coming in the ship with Clint Eastwood standing there watching it being real calm, it jumped to this romantic scene with this woman, then I was on the phone. But the part of it, I don't know where this came in, when I was at the bar eating lunch and I knew someone was going to die I believe it was at 4 o'clock and I told my friend and he believed me, like it was no surprise that I knew this. I was very matter-of-fact. The other part on the phone with my wife and the woman I was frustrated and angry that my wife would make such comments to this woman that weren't justified to this woman who had the same name as the woman who I went to high school with. That was a lot of years ago. She didn't look the same, she was attractive, she's very cute, but she wasn't the same as the

woman from high school, she just had the same name. It is
an unusual name, the only woman I have known with that
name.

This is another complex dream, with several scenes and a mixture of time references from present, future, and past. The dreamer does not express his anger at his wife's interference with his potential sex partner until the end of the dream. After the first scene, he dreams he has power to predict a death, and then projects that responsibility onto a calm (not angry) hero who observes the disaster. Then he returns to express his frustration and anger at his ex-wife.

It should be clear by now why, listening to these reports, I sometimes felt like the teacher in the Peanuts cartoon who is being consoled by the little girl reporting her complex dream. What we can say about the dreams of the control volunteers is that they introduce many characters and changes of scene. They combine older memory material with images from the present. They also demonstrate directly feelings about the former spouse. In the first, the dreamer enjoys excluding her ex-husband from her preparations for sexual attractiveness. In the second dream, the dreamer is angry about the ex-wife's interference with his potential sexual encounter with a new woman.

What a treasure these dreams are for appreciating the mind as it works away at an emotional issue. When no emotion is expressed, and there is no relation of current images to older memories, and when the dreamer's role in the dream story is passive, dreams of the former spouse appear to have no sustained impact on the waking mood disorder. After all, these are from dreamers who did not recover from the depression within the 5 months. The dreams of the two depressed women who would recover link the past and present, express strong feelings, and take actions that are appropriate to the dream situations they create. These dreams seem almost like a rehearsal for recovery; both women see the husband in a bad light and walk away.

Thus, the dream process that actively mediates the negative mood associated with some waking experience seems to have the effect of stabilizing a better morning mood, and that mood progressively improves at each testing point. The dreams illustrate how this takes place; in them, dreamers accept their need to move ahead, to leave the former spouse behind, and to initiate a change in their identities from married to that of effective single people. The dreams of those stuck in depression show no such movement. These are the depressed who will most likely need a therapeutic intervention, perhaps antidepressant medication or psychotherapy, or both, to overcome their depression.

Perhaps some day there will be an application for these research findings. Dream collection might become a screening tool useful in determining a patient's psychological resiliency. Dreams that fail to function as mood regulators within sleep and fail to initiate an adaptive change in the structure of the self system might serve to identify more quickly those who will require some professional help in order to function more effectively.

Sleepwalking into Danger: Murders | 5
Without Motives

Merciful powers!
Restrain in me the cursed thoughts that nature
Gives way to in repose.

—William Shakespeare, *Macbeth*

I served as a sleep expert for the trials of two landmark cases in which sleep-related aggression led to a charge of murder in the first degree. Both defense teams claimed that the act was carried out while the accused was in a nonconscious state and therefore not responsible for his actions. This was an especially difficult argument to make at the time (the first trial took place in 1990, the second in 1999). The methodology required to establish the validity of a non–rapid eye movement (NREM) sleepwalking violence diagnosis had not yet caught up with the need for it.

Although the two crimes had much in common, the defendants were two very different people. Ken Parks was in his early twenties, Scott Falater in his early forties. Ken had not finished high school and was unemployed; Scott had a degree in electrical engineering and was in middle management at a large firm. Ken was over his head in gambling debts, whereas Scott had a good income and no money problems. With only this basic description of the two men, it might have been expected that their trials would have the opposite outcome, but Ken was acquitted by a Canadian court while Scott was convicted and sentenced to life imprisonment without the possibility of parole. He is currently serving his sentence in Arizona. Although cases like these are rare, there is a long history of trials for sleep-related violence in which the accused was bewilderingly motiveless. Sleepwalking with violence is one of the parasomnia disorders of sleep. These violent events only occur in relation to sleep; the defendant is perfectly sane while awake. The attack occurs shortly after the sleeper has arisen, within the first hour or two of sleep. Although the behavior may look like waking, the person's mental state is more like sleep. This puts their diagnosis within the category of a sleep disorder.

I will review the Falater case in some detail to explain the disorder of sleep violence and what it adds to our understanding of the ways in which waking experiences impact sleeping behavior, and vice versa. This case is special because we have both an eye witness account and a wealth of dream material hand-written by Falater since his conviction, which he sent to me for 9 years during his incarceration. This presents a rare opportunity to follow the sleeping mind as it copes with the emotional aftermath of an act that dramatically changed a person's life and ended that of another. The incident took place in 1997, before the newest sleep diagnostic methods were developed, tested, and published to allow sleep specialists to differentiate sleepwalkers from those who do not meet the criteria for this sleep disorder. Scott Falater remains hopeful that a retrial will be granted on the grounds that this research, which could establish his diagnosis, was not available at the time of his conviction. What insight can this case provide into the mind deprived of normal, healthy sleep?

The Scott Falater Case: The Pool Pump Murder

There is no doubt that on January 16 1997, Scott Falater killed his wife. His neighbor, Greg Koons, was an eye witness. It was Koons who called 911 and who stood by until the police arrived. He led them to the scene and gave his account.

"It was at about 10:30 P.M. when I heard a commotion next door; dogs barking and a woman screaming. I was in bed at that time but not yet asleep. I got up to see what was going on." Greg described how he climbed up to look over the garden wall that separated his property from the Falater's backyard. There was a body lying next to the outdoor pool. "My first impression was that the noise must have come from a party and the body was likely someone who had passed out after having too much to drink." Then, he said he remembered, "these neighbors are Mormons, forbidden to drink."

Just then a light came on in a second-story window through which Greg could see Scott moving about from room to room. Shortly after that, Scott came outside, raised his hand to restrain his dogs from jumping up, and stood over the body with what Greg first described as "a blank staring look."

"Then he turned and walked into the garage." Pointing to the garage, Greg went on, "When he came out a short time later, he was drawing on a pair of heavy canvas gloves. He knelt by the body, dragged it to the edge of the pool, and rolled it into the water. At first I thought he was trying to revive the person. Then I realized he must be drowning them." At that point, Koons had seen enough. He left his post and hurried inside to call for help.

Soon there was the sound of sirens approaching the quiet suburban street. Several cars pulled up, doors opened, and paramedics, uniformed police, and a photographer assembled. Greg met them and led them to the backyard. The photographer went to work documenting the scene. Others pulled the body from the bloody pool water. The officer in charge ordered a search of the grounds looking for evidence and for the person, or persons, involved.

While all this was going on, Scott reports he was sound asleep in the upstairs bedroom he shared with his wife. He woke abruptly to the sounds of dogs barking and voices below his window. Was it an intruder? He jumped up and was halfway down the stairs when the police charged in through the back door and met him. One of the officers, his gun drawn, shouted: "Get down on the floor. Face down. Hands behind the back." Scott was handcuffed and questioned. "How many people are in the house?" He answered that there were four people in the house, meaning himself, his wife, and their son and daughter. Scott did not know then that his wife Yarmila was lying outside, dead from 44 stab wounds. The children, Megan and Michael, were still asleep in their beds. They had slept through all the commotion.

Scott was marched out of the house and placed in the back seat of a squad car parked at the curb. The neighbors had begun to gather and line the sidewalk opposite the house, watching and speculating about what was going on. Scott sat in the car, puzzled. Through the partially open car window he overheard scraps of conversation. From these he learned that his wife was hurt. He wondered how badly, why he was left in the car, and why no one had told him what was happening. Were they searching for an intruder? Were his kids all right? Why was he handcuffed? A long hour passed before he was driven to the police station, where a formal videotaped interrogation began. A detective asked Scott over and over, "What set you off? Why did you kill your wife?" Scott sat slumped in a corner, crushed and baffled. He asked, "Why do you think I am the one responsible?" The detective pointed out to him that he had blood on his neck and a fresh bandage on one hand. Scott looked at his hand, puzzled. He could not answer any of the detective's questions. He had, and still has, no memory of what had taken place between the time he fell into bed, dead tired around 9:45 P.M., and when he woke up to the sounds of the police entering his house. What happened during that interval, when his wife was killed and Scott was seen rolling her body into their backyard pool, was pieced together from the neighbor's report and the deductions of the police. Scott knew nothing of this at the time, and even now can add no facts nor supply any explanation to account for what happened. His only explanation to himself at the time, he told me, was that he must have been going crazy.

Was He Crazy?

Was Scott's murder of his wife the result of a psychotic episode, a type of dissociation disorder, or perhaps of an epileptic attack, a temporal lobe or complex partial seizure? Scott was examined by a psychiatrist who found him to be depressed over his wife's death, but any serious psychiatric disorder that would provide an explanation for the killing was ruled out. The court ordered a battery of psychological tests, which were interpreted as being within normal limits. I reviewed these myself and agreed with the analysis. Scott's profile on the Minnesota Multiphasic Personality Inventory (MMPI), a test widely used as a diagnostic instrument to determine the degree and type of various psychopathological tendencies, was not only normal, it was without peaks of disturbance in any specific area. A neurologist examined Scott and cleared him of having a seizure disorder. He was declared to be in excellent health.

A prominent legal firm was engaged to defend Scott. The lawyers first turned their attention toward finding some motive for the killing, but they were baffled. The Falaters had had no financial trouble and no marital problems. Everyone interviewed offered the same opinion: The Falaters were an ideal couple. They had married young and after 20 years were still in love. Scott had a good income and a secure middle-management position in a large corporation where he had recently been promoted and put in charge of an important project. The children, both teenagers, were well behaved, smart, and did well in school. The family was described as loving and close; disagreements were few according to the children, and differences of opinion were settled by discussion. Recently they had considered moving to a larger house in a better neighborhood they were now able to afford, but they had decided to stay where they were, in an economically and ethnically diverse neighborhood, so that the children would continue to have friends of many different backgrounds. Scott had no police record and had never been violent. His family members and both children described him as even-tempered, a man of good will, an elder in his church who, with his wife, did good works in the community.

The only curious issue that surfaced after long hours of investigation was that Scott had not been sleeping well for the previous few months. He was going through a prolonged period of stress over a decision that he found hard to make. The big project he had been given at work was to develop a new computer chip, and it was not going well. Scott had felt excited by the opportunity but now worried that his company was starting too late, that the competition was too far ahead for them to succeed. The pressure was significant, but he had realized that he was probably not going to succeed. Scott felt morally obligated to tell the management that, in his opinion, they should cut their losses and close down the project. What stopped him was his fear that he would be seen as a failure who could not live up to their expectations. This was hard for him to admit. Competence in his work was a major part of Scott's self-concept, and a source of pride. Shutting down the project might also jeopardize the team that had been assembled to help him, and who looked up to him as their leader. He hated to be responsible for their job failures as well.

And so Scott procrastinated, putting off taking action from week to week. He could not sleep well with this problem on his mind. To fight off the resulting fatigue and to stay alert at meetings, he began to use caffeine tablets during the day. He stuck to his usual routine of getting up early each morning to teach a group of teenagers at his church before heading to his office to face the ever-present dilemma: Should he keep trying or should he confess failure, letting down those who had put their faith in him?

When Sleep Turns Violent

Once the medical and psychiatric experts had ruled out other explanations for Scott's attack on Yarmila, the idea that the stabbing was the result of a sleep disorder was considered. Scott's sister Laura suggested this possibility. She could not believe that Scott would harm Yarmila intentionally. There had to be some logical explanation. She began a computer search for similar cases, eventually finding the Ken Parks case that had occurred ten years earlier. The two homicides had much in common. Ken Parks had arisen from sleep, driven to his mother-in-law's home, and stabbed her to death. He was acquitted by a jury on the grounds that he was sleepwalking. In the Canadian court, Ken's actions were referred to as a "noninsane automatism." The fact that Ken too had been asleep for a short time before the fatal attack reminded Laura of Scott's sleepwalking as a child, and that he still had occasional episodes. She had a vivid memory of one instance during which she was the one who had been hurt. It had happened shortly before he was married. Scott was 20 then, 2 years older than his sister, and still living at home. About midnight, Laura was in the kitchen fixing something to eat when Scott came downstairs in his pajamas and headed for the back door. She said she recognized that he was sleepwalking from the blank, staring look on his face. She stepped quickly between him and the kitchen door to block his way. He grabbed her by the shoulders and threw her across the room. She landed hard on her tailbone. His roughness startled her, because it was so unlike his usual behavior. Laura wondered if sleepwalking could explain what had happened. It was at least a strong possibility. Scott's lawyers agreed.

The idea that he might have been sleepwalking had not occurred to Scott, and he resisted it. He was a practical-minded man and, as an electrical engineer, not given to flights of fantasy. Although the notion did not seem plausible to him, Scott's legal team decided to make sleepwalking the central argument of his defense. They would need experts to give their opinions, and that was when they contacted me. I had served as an expert for the defense in the Ken Parks case, the one Laura had found on the internet. In the Parks case, the decision to acquit was appealed by the Crown (prosecution), but the acquittal was upheld by the Supreme Court of Canada. The basis for the high court's opinion was that this was such an unusual set of circumstances that they were highly unlikely to ever be repeated. I read that decision as I considered agreeing to be a sleep expert in the Falater case.

Sleepwalking is so common in young children that pediatricians, if consulted at all, usually just reassure parents that it will pass eventually. For the most part, they are right; sleepwalking rarely persists into adulthood. When it does, it is much more common in men than in women. While youngsters who sleepwalk are rarely violent, in a very large telephone survey study, 2.1% of adults reported they were currently violent during their sleep.

Separate from sleepwalking but related to it is another sleep disorder known as *sleep terrors*. A child with sleep terrors typically sits up abruptly and screams as if terrified; he may just fall back asleep or he may run about in a glassy-eyed frenzy of escape-like activity, with a very high heart rate. If a parent attempts to control and console the child, he will stay stiff and distraught, and may even turn on the comforter and beat that person with his fists. When children are little, this behavior is harmless; but experience has yielded some sound advice: "Take care before interfering with a sleepwalker."

Sleep terror attacks happen in the first hours of sleep. Although they look very dramatic, they are not caused by bad dreams and leave no memory behind in the morning. They are *NREM parasomnias*, one of a family of sleep problems first named "disorders of arousal" by Roger Broughton, a Canadian neurologist and sleep researcher. These disorders occur in roughly 15%–30% of all youngsters at a specific time of night and stage of sleep. They happen within the first 1–3 hours of the night, when the child's first deep sleep cycle is very long and delta waves are high and slow. Sleep terrors appear to be a disorder associated with rapid physical growth and with the development of the neurological networks sustaining new learning. Once this growth is largely accomplished, the proportion of slow-wave sleep (SWS) gradually reduces through adolescence, and the correlated sleepwalking and sleep terrors also slowly fade away.

According to the scenario the police put together to explain his activity on the night his wife was killed, Scott engaged in a complicated series of behaviors over an extended period of time. The police believed he got up from sleep and walked safely downstairs and out to the garage, where he changed into work clothes, took his tools from the trunk of his car, and went to finish repairing a pump that filtered water for the backyard pool. Yarmila had asked him to do this when he came home from work that evening. He had wanted to talk over his work problem with her, but put that off until dinner was over. He then told her he intended to tell the administrators at his office that the project needed to be terminated. Yarmila advised him not to do this. "Just tell them what they want to hear," was her conclusion. Scott was disappointed, and told me that he responded that he had gone along long enough. The couple ended the conversation at that point, both feeling dissatisfied. They washed the dinner dishes and watched TV together while the children did their homework. When the children went up to bed at about 9 o'clock, Scott went outside to inspect the pool project. He remembers thinking, "At least I can do this job." He determined that an O-ring needed to be replaced, but it was stuck. He worked on the project for about half an hour but he was tired, and it soon became too dark to finish. Inside, Yarmila was still on the couch watching television. He kissed her good night and headed for bed. That was at about 9:30 P.M. Scott remembers that he put on his pajama pants but left his tee shirt on, and then fell soundly asleep. That was his last memory before awaking to the noise of the police entering his house.

Since it was 10:30 when the neighbor heard the commotion next door, the police reasoned that Scott must have gotten up between 10 and 10:15 and gone back outside, intent on finishing the pool pump project. His tools were not found by the pool but in a Tupperware container in the wheel well of his car, along with a blood-stained knife and bloody work clothes. Since Scott was no longer visible when Greg Koons went to see what the noise was about, Scott must have put on his work clothes earlier and worked for a short while, perhaps using the knife to pry out the stubborn O-ring. The police suggested that Yarmila may have heard her husband go out the patio door and likely followed him in order to bring him back inside. If she touched him while he was bent down working, it likely startled him, and this was probably when she was attacked. Scott then changed from his work clothes, put them and his tools away, and went upstairs. He missed washing the blood from his neck, put a bandage on his hand, and went back down to the pool site where Koons saw him standing over the body. He then rolled it into the pool before going upstairs again and back to bed.

Since neither Greg Koons nor the police witnessed the stabbing of Yarmila, just how that happened is pure conjecture. The shift in behavior from the benign repair activity to an act of aggression has been known to happen when a sleepwalker misperceives a harmless gesture to be an attack, for which the appropriate response is to fight back. Sleepwalkers have no awareness of who they are harming. They do not recognize faces while in this peculiar brain state.

Before I agreed to help with the defense in the earlier Ken Parks case, I had not treated many adult sleepwalkers as patients. I had worked with some youngsters who had scared their parents by getting out of the house while sleepwalking. One was found in pajamas and bare feet directing traffic on a snowy night in Chicago. The police brought him home. Another youngster walked in pajamas to the house of a friend at midnight, then rang their bell. The startled parents walked him home. This boy grew up and attended medical college, reintroducing himself to me following lecture I gave to his freshman class. I was happy to hear his sleepwalking nights were behind him.

I had also treated a few adults who had hurt themselves while in a sleepwalking state, but none who had been aggressive toward others. I welcomed the chance to learn more. I began to prepare by reading what literature I could find on the subject, discovering many accounts of cases like that of Ken Parks dating back some 400 years. In one, a sleeping woman threw her baby out a window, believing the house to be on fire. In another, a man hit his wife with a shovel, thinking she was a beast attacking him. Most often, these reports appeared in legal journals as a single unusual case report, followed by a discussion about the degree of criminal responsibility the perpetrator should bear for such an act.

The most helpful article I found was written in 1974, by a Canadian psychiatrist, Dr. Alexander Bonkalo, who summarized the common threads that marked these acts as being symptoms of a sleep disorder rather than a psychiatric condition. Best of all, Bonkalo listed a set of guidelines for determining whether an act of aggression had likely happened while the perpetrator was in a state of nonconscious awareness. Checking the Ken Parks case against this list, I felt he matched the sleepwalking criteria. Later, I tested the facts of Scott Falater's case against the same points. Bonkalo's criteria have now been largely adopted as the basis for making a diagnosis of sleepwalking disorder by the psychiatric handbook, the *Diagnostic and Statistical Manual of Mental Disorders* (DSM IV-TR) and by the *International Classification of Sleep Disorders* (ICSD) in the diagnostic manual of the American Academy of Sleep Medicine.

The Diagnosis of Sleepwalking

The first and most important fact to establish is *when* the arousal into sleep-walking activity takes place. The arousal must be from NREM sleep, and it must occur at the beginning of the night's sleep—most often, this is in the first period of SWS, in the first third of the night. Scott Falater had started up to bed at about 9:30 P.M. He was seen by the neighbor at about 10:45 P.M., sometime after the stabbing and his departure from the scene. When he returned, Greg Koons observed him standing over a body, which he then rolled into the pool. Greg's call to the police was recorded at 10:58. This suggests that, if Scott had fallen asleep immediately, before he had fully changed into his pajamas, he must have gotten up to continue the pool repair after he had been sleeping for less than an hour. This would place the timing of his arousal within the first NREM sleep cycle, before he had reached REM sleep and any dreaming.

The second important item in Bonkalo's list of criteria concerns whether the person has any *memory* of the event. Scott could recall nothing of the events between falling into bed at about 9:30 P.M. and waking up to the noise of the police entering his house. Not only had he no recall of what happened between these two periods; he still has no memory of it, even today. This was also true of Ken Parks, who asked me if there was a way I could help him get back his memory of that period, perhaps through hypnosis. I asked him gently, "Would you want that?" He hung his head for a few moments and said, "Only if you could take it away again."

Next, there must be no attempt to *cover up* the attack. Although Scott had changed out of his bloody work clothes, put them and his tools away, and gone upstairs and washed up, he did not clean the blood from the knife, nor did he dispose of his bloodstained work clothes or remove blood from his neck. What struck me as most important was that he did not hide the body. It was left in plain view floating in their pool. This was not the act of a man in full possession of his decision-making powers.

In a previous murder case studied in our Sleep Center, I had refused to testify on behalf of the defendant based on his cover-up behavior. The wife of the accused had been out for the evening with friends. When she returned home around midnight, her husband had been asleep for about an hour, and was probably in deep sleep. She playfully jumped on top of him. He was startled by what he perceived as an attack by a stranger.

Anyone awakened abruptly from deep sleep is initially a bit confused. If the phone rings in the middle of the night, it takes a minute or more for us to recognize who is calling and what he or she is talking about. This is called "sleep inertia," and it lasts longer when the arousal is from SWS than it does from REM. In this case, the accused was a tall man with great muscular arm strength. He threw his wife off the bed and jumped down after her. They got tangled in the bedclothes at the foot of the bed. While still in the dark, he got her in a choke hold and strangled her. He then ran to check on his children. Finding them still asleep, he returned to his bedroom and uncovered the body. He told me that when he recognized his wife, he sat on the side of the bed and cried. Then he carried her out to his car, placed her in the trunk, and drove out of town. He abandoned the car and walked home.

After four nights of sleep testing, we could not establish a sleepwalking diagnosis in this case. On one of those nights, in the hopes of precipitating an arousal, I instructed our head tech to wait through the first hour of deep sleep, and then to throw a pillowcase full of books onto the sleeper's chest to simulate the event that had resulted in his wife's death. The tech did as requested, but the sleeper woke up fully conscious, then rolled over, and went back to sleep. The killing of his wife was most likely a case of sleep inertia, confusion on being aroused from deep sleep by what he interpreted as an "attack." He quickly regained full consciousness and acted rationally by checking on his kids and attempting to cover up his unintended lethal attack. I could not support this as a sleep disorder. He was tried and convicted.

The fourth point on the Bonkalo list of sleepwalking violence criteria is *unresponsiveness* during the episode. Scott did not respond to his wife's screams, which were loud enough to be heard by the neighbor, nor did he awaken from his mixed state of consciousness/unconsciousness when he held her head under the cold pool water. He did not seem to "see" Koons looking at him over the wall. His senses of hearing, touch, and vision (for face recognition) were all somewhat impaired. Ken Parks also failed to hear his mother-in-law's screams, which woke and frightened the children sleeping upstairs. He did not appear to feel the pain from the serious injuries to his hands caused by his victim as she tried to defend herself with a kitchen knife, nor did he recognize his victim when he said he "woke up" over the body of a woman with a "help me" look.

Well into the police interview with Ken Parks, the transcript indicates that he said, "Hey, my hands hurt." He was then transported to a hospital and a hand surgeon was summoned from his sleep to come and do an extensive repair. Both the Parks case and the Falater case met Bonkalo's fourth qualification.

Next on Bonkalo's list is the importance of *ruling out other explanations*; that the lethal attack is not the result of substance abuse or a medical condition. Scott did not drink alcohol nor use illegal drugs. He was cleared of any medical condition, and no alcohol or other substances were found in the urine screening test done when he was first arrested. Nothing was found that might have been a trigger for this behavior. The possible role of his recent use of the caffeine tablets to fight off daytime sleepiness was not noted to be of any importance upon his arrest.

The next question is whether the sleepwalker shows *profound remorse* over the death they caused. The psychiatrist who examined Scott reported that he was devastated by the loss of his wife. He cried silently while talking with me and again during the trial, when photos of his wife's body were shown. He did not wipe away the tears, nor did he allow himself to sob audibly. Scott's control came from his belief that "God knows that my heart is pure." Ken Parks was also deeply depressed. Repeated personality testing showed high "D" scores, and I confirmed this in my interactions with him before his trial. He asked me then, "Why would I do that when I had everything to lose and nothing to gain?" A very good question.

Bonkalo then stresses the importance of determining whether there is a *genetic basis* for the sleepwalking disorder. Does the person have a history of sleepwalking as a child, or a strong family history of this problem? Scott had both. A court-ordered family tree was constructed, and it showed that many members of the family had had episodes of sleepwalking, bed wetting after the age of 5, and sleep terrors. The tree was heavy with sleep disorders; Scott's son Michael was also a sleepwalker.

Bonkalo's last point is that the attack makes *no rational sense*. In the Falater murder case, even the very diligent prosecutor could not establish any motivation for the attack. He tried out many possibilities. He proposed the idea that Yarmila wanted more children and Scott did not; that she had put on weight and was not as trim as she was as a bride; that Yarmila was not as committed to the Church of the Latter Day Saints as was Scott. None of these theories could be established as fact. All were denied by the family and friends who testified. And none seemed strong enough, even if true, to support a motive for murder.

To Bonkalo's list of sleepwalking violence signs, I added one more, based on my review of previous cases. Adult sleepwalkers are able to find their way in space without trouble. They do not fumble about as youngsters do. Scott went downstairs to the garage, changed into work clothes, got his tools, and went to work. I had encountered instances of clothing changes in many other cases; one man told me he knew when he had been sleepwalking only when he found muddy clothes carefully put away in his bureau the next morning. Complex motor behaviors, too, are common to adult sleepwalkers. Ken Parks drove his car without incident to his in-laws' home some 23 kilometers away, where the aggression took place. What true sleepwalkers cannot do is recognize the faces of those they attack, even loved ones. These two visual pathways, one for space localization and the other for face recognition, terminate in different areas in the brain. Perhaps, as the police suggested, Yarmila startled Scott with her touch when she went outside to lead her husband back to bed. In the mixed brain state of partial waking and partial sleep, he did not recognize her and attacked her with the knife he was using to pry out the worn O-ring. This event, horrendous as it was, left no memory for Scott—a blank spot remains. When Scott awakened to the noise of the police, he was beyond the SWS time and so regained full consciousness. He has a full memory of the rest of that night's events.

At this point in my thinking, after having read all I could find about sleepwalking violence in order to participate in the Parks case, and having examined all the material collected for the Falater case, I felt I needed a reality check of my own. I asked Scott's defense lawyers to arrange for sleep studies to be done at a local hospital, and to set up a meeting for me with the defendant. I wanted to find out if I would believe him when he told me his story. I needed to judge whether he had remained in a state of confusion for some time after the stabbing, as he cleaned up, came back to the body, and rolled her into the pool, before going back to bed. This constituted not one aggressive act but two—the abrupt stabbing and the delayed drowning. This became a stumbling point for the jury when Scott came to trial. I myself had never encountered that scenario. There were no cases like it in the sleep or forensic literature, although much about these strange disorders was then and still is unknown.

A point of contention is just how long a state of confusional arousal lasts after a sleepwalking aggression takes place. The literature suggests this is a short period of about 15 minutes. Following the stabbing of his mother-in-law, Ken Parks was not fully conscious even as he drove to the police station and announced that he thought he "may have killed some people." Scott Falater also seemed to remain in a state of semiconsciousness for well over an hour after the initial attack.

My first impression of Scott when he met with me at the lockup where he was being held was that he looked to be rather a cool customer, but at the same time truly bewildered by the circumstances that had brought him there.

He knew that the facts pointed to his guilt, but with no memory of what had happened, he had no sense of owning the experience. He did not appear to be in a state of distress as we shook hands. A slightly balding, serious-looking man dressed in his prison jumpsuit, he was a bit of a nerd, I thought. We circled around one another, getting acquainted, until I asked him what he thought would happen to him as a result of the trial to come. He calmly explained his view. "There are only two possibilities and both are acceptable to me. If I will be found guilty," he said "I will receive the death penalty. If that is the case I will rejoin Yarmila in heaven because God knows that my heart is pure and He will allow us to be together. Or, I will be acquitted, in which case I will be able to raise my children and go on with my life."

Scott's faith and his logical mind were sustaining him. He did not consider a third possibility: A life sentence without any possibility of parole. Under these circumstances, he could neither raise his children nor be with Yarmila. As we talked of this, tears began to flow, and I saw the man beneath the control. "What upsets me the most," he said quietly, "is that I didn't know I was killing her, but she did." He explained this further. "She must have looked right at me and wondered how I, who loved her, could be attacking her." After a few quiet moments, he said softly, "She was my best friend and the only woman I ever loved."

The trial attracted a good deal of media attention. I waited to be called to testify sitting next to another defense witness, the head technician from another sleep lab that had done an independent scoring of Scott's 4 nights of sleep studies. Reporters from the local papers loitered, hoping to pick up scraps of information from witnesses as they left the courtroom. Although I declined to comment, a photographer took my picture. The prosecutor used this incident to accuse me of "grandstanding" for the press.

When I was sworn in, I was aware that the jury did not seem sympathetic. They did not appear to take my expert testimony seriously, sitting back in their seats; one rolled her eyes. A single juror, an elderly black man, leaned forward and followed my testimony closely. Aside from him, the jurors looked as if they had already made up their minds. The prosecutor was sarcastic and dismissive of the concept of "sleepwalking," and he attacked me and my motives, implying I was testifying for money. I was happy to tell him I was offering my services *pro bono*.

The prosecution produced its own sleep expert, who made a strong case that Scott had not been sleepwalking when he killed Yarmila. He argued that Scott had never gone to sleep, before or after the attack, and therefore that he was fully responsible for Yarmila's death. He based his argument on the belief that Scott had behaved logically. He had washed up afterwards, had put on a bandage, and had returned to the body and committed a further act of aggression by holding Yarmila's head under water. According to this expert, Scott's behavior demonstrated that he had a clear memory of what had happened; after all, he was able to return to the body because he knew where it was. He argued that Scott had not gone back to sleep after the "second murder" but likely was on his way back to the scene to clean up further, and perhaps to dispose of the body, when the police arrived. This expert went on to claim that Scott had planned the murder, citing the fact that the Tupperware container, where the police had found the bloody work clothes and knife, had been newly purchased. This alone indicated conscious planning. The jury agreed; this alternative scenario was apparently easier to believe at the time than was a sleepwalking defense. Jurors told reporters after the trial that, although no motive had been established for the murder, the accused must have had "unconscious hostility" toward his wife, which drove him to kill her.

I had testified before the prosecution's sleep expert, and I was required to leave the courtroom after my time on the stand. I was given no opportunity to respond to the other expert's argument, which to me seemed a hypothetical conjecture—an attempt to explain a nonrational, unconscious act as logical, conscious behavior.

As I was packing my notes into my briefcase and preparing to leave, the very large uniformed bailiff who had stood in the courtroom throughout the trial came over and asked me if I had a business card. I handed one over and asked him what his interest was. He looked a little abashed and said, "I beat people up in my sleep." Here was another violent sleepwalker confessing to a disorder that the jury had not found believable in Scott's case.

Sleep Studies as Evidence

What about the sleep studies that had been performed on Scott at a local hospital? What did they show? Four all-night recordings had been conducted. On none of the nights did Scott attempt to get up early on, when SWS should predominate. (Unfortunately, he was wearing iron shackles locked to the bed, which alone would have inhibited motor activity.) What the study did show was Scott had almost no deep sleep; in fact, he had brief arousals throughout all of his sleep. Most of these were clustered in the first 2 hours of the night. By the time these tests were done, long after Yarmila's killing in January, Scott's state of mind and his sleep had changed significantly. His sleep was anything but solid; it was very easily disrupted, but this disruption might well be understood as a result of his awareness of the importance of the sleep test findings to his case. One cannot will oneself into having SWS, but anxiety might well produce a fitful night. Also, at Scott's age, SWS is greatly reduced in males. I argued this point during the trial, but it led only to what observers felt was a dispute between the "so-called experts."

Since sleepwalking as a disorder is episodic, it is difficult to capture in a laboratory setting. When no behavioral arousal occurs during the test, standard sleep scoring of the sleepwalker does not differ from those of normal sleepers. At the time of Scott's trial, no distinctive signature had been found, nothing special in the brain waves, or timing of the first REM, to distinguish sleepwalkers from non-sleepwalkers. Only recently, beginning with publications in 2000, researchers developed two new ways to establish a sleepwalking diagnosis from sleep laboratory studies. The first involves a better way to elicit an arousal episode under laboratory circumstances in those with an established history of sleepwalking. The second is a more sophisticated analysis of the sleeper's brain waves.

The first involves a new protocol requiring two sleep studies. A standard diagnostic recording is made to rule out any other sleep disorder, followed by a period of 25 hours of sleep deprivation (the subject is kept awake all day and all night in the lab). A second recording then is performed during 7 hours of recovery sleep. When we are deprived of all sleep, it is SWS that shows an increase first, so this protocol was designed to increase the pressure for SWS, mimicking the effect of the chronic loss that typically precedes an adult sleepwalking event. Ken Parks had been sleeping badly for months, worrying about his gambling debts, and Scott Falater was anxious about his failure to solve the problem assigned to him at work.

Sleep deprivation alone has not proven to be a successful maneuver for provoking sleepwalking in the laboratory—an arousing stimulus must be added. The new protocol, designed too late to be of help to Scott, employs the sounding of increasingly louder tones, repeated until the sleeper responds. In those with a strong sleepwalking history, this method has worked remarkably well; furthermore, it has not resulted in any abnormal arousals in non-sleepwalker control subjects. The study that tested this protocol, published in 2008, reported that 100% of sleepwalkers (and none of the controls) experienced one or more sleepwalking events during the recovery sleep following 25 hours of sleep deprivation. These motor arousals are documented on video tape. Scott had served 2 years of his life term in a penitentiary when these results were reported.

The new diagnostic sleep protocol, which employs a period of sleep deprivation followed by a recovery night with auditory tones of increasing loudness, provokes the sleepwalking behavior—but it does not explain the mechanism involved. Several sets of research findings must be considered together to help clarify the underlying pathology. Earlier genetic work has found that known sleepwalkers have a particular genetic abnormality that makes them more easily aroused from SWS, but the same genetic marker was found more frequently in narcoleptic patients and those with REM behavior disorder as well. The single brain imaging study conducted on a sleepwalker *while sleepwalking* indicated that, during the sleepwalk, the young man did not shift into full consciousness—the brain areas associated with higher mental processes like judgment and reality-testing were under-activated.

The second recent breakthrough for diagnosing sleepwalking in the laboratory was originally reported as a more sophisticated method of scoring sleeping brain waves, using spectral analysis or power-density scoring. This technique counts the brain waves characteristic of each sleep stage according to their frequency and amplitude. When applied to the recordings of sleepwalkers, this method has revealed a consistently lower activity of delta waves in the first sleep cycle than in healthy controls. These findings have been replicated in studies done in three different laboratories in three different countries. This may be the missing evidence of a specific neurological flaw.

Sleepwalking Triggers

A childhood history of sleepwalking, and a family tree full of relatives with inadequate suppression of motor behavior during SWS in the first hour of the night, is not enough to cause a sleepwalking episode. Rather, it takes several coinciding conditions to make sleepwalking happen. A genetic heritage and a period of sleep loss (often due to emotional distress) are two of those conditions. An important third ingredient is the trigger.

A *sleepwalking trigger* is something that interferes with the natural drive to achieve more SWS following sleep deprivation. This stimulus propels the sleepwalker out of bed while still in a state of semiconsciousness. Several triggers are known to have this effect, although some are controversial. The first, as reported by many sleepwalkers, is some alerting noise. This has been incorporated into the laboratory test to induce a sleepwalking event following a period of sleep deprivation, as part of the new sleep study protocol. The authors of that study reported that, in trying to trigger a sleepwalking episode, they tested recovery sleep alone and sleep with increasingly loud tones alone. Neither worked nearly as well as both together. It took increased SWS plus tones of increasing volume to elicit the sleepwalking arousals in the laboratory. It appears that all sleepwalking triggers that work act as an opposing arousing force to prior sleep deprivation, which causes the brain to push for more SWS. Auditory tones force an arousal in the sleeper, as does the intake of excessive caffeine, sleep medications such as Ambien (because it has the effect of consolidating sleep, but at the same time lightens SWS), excessive alcohol, and some antipsychotic and antidepressant medications. All have the same effect of making the sleeper more easily aroused from SWS, especially when following a period of sleep deprivation. We know from power-density scoring that the amount of slow wave activity is abnormally low in sleepwalkers, even on nights when no prior sleep deprivation or sleepwalking has taken place. This means that we now have a sleep marker that will discriminate a sleepwalker from a non-sleepwalker—even when the sleepwalker has not actually walked during the sleep study. (Hot dog and thank goodness was my response to this news.)

In some adult sleepwalking cases, and more often in children, another potential trigger is the presence of a breathing disorder of sleep, *sleep apnea*. Sleep apnea leads to many brief arousals from sleep in sleepwalkers and non-sleepwalkers alike. The difference for those with a sleepwalking history is that repeated pauses in breathing do not just interrupt sleep; they provide the final push that propels the sleeper out of bed in *a confused state of mind*. In small children who snore and sleepwalk, a tonsillectomy has resolved both problems in many cases. Those sleepers who have been sleeping poorly over an extended period of time, which leads to a build-up of pressure for more deep sleep, and then ingest a substance that lightens this sleep, experience a loss of oxygen due to obstructed breathing, or are roused by a sudden noise are likely to have a confused behavioral sleepwalk. In Scott's case, the final trigger may well have been the caffeine tablets to which, as a practicing Mormon, his system was naïve.

The loss of sleep that precedes a sleepwalking episode is not the same as that typical of insomnia. The sleepwalker's many arousals, which delay their transition into REM sleep, also puts off dreaming. When sleepwalkers are aroused from sleep, it is at a specific time within the first third of the night, and they are brought to their feet in a mixed sleep/wake brain state, one which allows complex motor behaviors to take place without rational control. What behavior then takes place seems to depend on what was on the sleeper's mind, and on which basic drive was in a heightened state, before sleep—and is still active during the first hour of sleep. This may be a drive for food, for sex, to escape from danger, to strike out against someone misperceived as an enemy, or just to explore new territory. Roughly, we can call these basic survival drives.

In Scott's case, there was the ongoing anxiety of having to admit his failure at work to produce the chip he had been assigned to develop. This laid the groundwork for many nights of unrefreshing sleep. Then, two new events heightened his disturbed state. He told his wife that he was going to report to upper management that the project should be terminated, and she advised him to "just tell them what they want to hear." Their difference of opinion on what was the right thing to do was still unresolved when he went to bed. The second source of internal tension for Scott was the malfunctioning pool filter motor that his wife had asked him to fix. Here was something easy for him, given his engineering skills. He worked on the project before going to bed but did not complete it, promising himself that he would do it later. He went to sleep with these two irritants still active: Yarmila had not supported his decision to admit his failure at work, and he had not done the simple repair she requested. Would this generate enough hostility to cause him to stab her to death if he were in a rational state of mind? Hardly; but, given his state of sleep deprivation, Scott was being driven to produce more SWS, and the caffeine tablets he had taken were having the opposite effect. They were making him more easily aroused from the first sleep hour, but not in a clear conscious state. In rising to fix the pool pump, Scott set out to put one of these tensions to rest in order to restore his image of himself as competent at his work and a good husband. When Yarmila interrupted that work, his drive to repair his self-esteem by completing the simple job was blocked. Blind as he was then as to who was standing in his way, his reaction was swift and strong. This is my conjecture about the psychology of the attack. It is, of course, unproven and not provable, but neither is the scenario of his being awake offered by the prosecutor's sleep expert. My interpretation fits with what I know of Scott Falater and of his personality and values.

Scott remains in the penitentiary. Meanwhile, there have been more cases in the courts and more research. Most exciting are the new findings that allow a better diagnostic certainty in the sleep laboratory. Scott's case is illustrative of the need to understand sleep abnormalities within the context of the whole person, the self system of organized traits and values, the emotional structures people bring to interpretation of their waking experiences, and the present state of their emotional economy. The actions of those suffering from a NREM parasomnia give us the opportunity to study behavior when it is unleashed from the constraints of reality while we sleep. Scott, over-controlled in his emotional expression, a perfectionist, and driven to do good work, had exhausted himself attempting to hold on course the task he had been given. When he could no longer sleep nor solve his work problem, he turned to Yarmila for support and she let him down. If he had been able to stay asleep and get into REM, perhaps he might have been able to down-regulate his frustrated emotional state in dreams, progressively from REM to REM throughout the night. Her husband's sleep deprivation plus excessive caffeine use, on top of his vulnerable sleep system, was a lethal mix for Yarmila.

I vowed to continue to do what I could to secure a retrial on the basis of new research that had not been available at the time of Scott's trial. His lawyers drew up a petition partly based on material I supplied from research papers. The same judge who sentenced him rejected this appeal. It was turned down, I expect, because the sleep expert who testified for the prosecution wrote a rebuttal stating that the new research had not been confirmed in other independent laboratories. Actually the distinctive low SWS activity of sleepwalkers had been replicated in three different labs at that time. That sleep expert also repeated his argument that Scott had not been sleepwalking at the time but was wide awake, and so fully responsible for his wife's death.

The appeal for a new trial moved to the next level, the state Supreme Court, which also rejected it. There is now no place to address a further appeal except at the federal level. This being the last hope, Scott's lawyers are moving slowly. They plan to wait for more support in the research literature and for more open-minded judges to be appointed. Meanwhile, many other cases have come to trial, and some of these defendants have been acquitted. I credit this change partly to the increased publicity about these incidents, and the acceptance of the idea that some people have a genuine sleep disorder that results in strange nocturnal behaviors. This is not as exotic a notion now as it was at the time of Scott's trial. Journalists have hopped on these cases as interesting stories, and frequently seek comments from professionals with sleep expertise. Several prominent sleep research professionals have refused to be involved in any criminal case in which disordered sleep is implicated. Some have justified this in position papers that make logical sense; their claim is that, even if a person is a sleepwalker by history and this is confirmed by laboratory evaluation, one can never know or prove with absolute certainty that the person was sleepwalking *at the time the criminal behavior occurred*. This position has reduced the willingness of some sleep disorder services even to evaluate these patients.

I disagree with this position. I believe that if we have specialized knowledge that can be applied to determine whether someone who is charged meets the diagnostic criteria of a NREM parasomnia, then it is consistent with the ethics of our profession to offer our informed opinion on the likelihood that the act in question is or is not compatible with this diagnosis. That is all that an expert witness is required to do. This is an arguable point, and it is currently being strongly debated. Certainly, testifying in open court is not a walk in the park, especially when such trials are set up to be adversarial in nature, with dueling experts and one-upmanship rather than truth-seeking opportunities. I came away from the Falater trial with new information and motivation to continue trying to make sense out of the mind in sleep. Were the jurors right who assumed that Scott had "unconscious hostility" toward his wife? If so, where and how could we find evidence of this? Freud would say in his dreams. After the trial, Scott thanked me for my efforts on his behalf and in his characteristic way asked what he could do for me in return. I asked him to keep a dream diary and to send it to me. He has done this more or less regularly on a monthly basis ever since. I now have almost 200 hand-written dream reports from Scott, accompanied by a letter that provides context of his waking experiences in the penitentiary, and how he is managing. His first letters were written with the stub of a pencil while he was on suicide precautions in solitary confinement.

Let us now turn to Scott's dreams for some insight into how his sleeping mind might have been picturing his wife. Given that many years have passed since his arrest, and that his waking life is now full of other challenges, what can we hope to learn? Scott has provided a large sample of dreams, written out over a period of almost 9 years. This makes it possible to identify stable elements that define his self-concept, and to examine what motivates him and how he organizes emotion-evoking events.

If this were a formal research study, it would be full of hazards. Has Scott censored his reports and given me only those dreams that show him at his best? I do not think so, given the dream reports themselves. Can I be an unbiased judge of these data, since I strongly hope to see Scott retried at least, and if possible, released for time served? I have done my best to treat these objectively by counting specific elements. What hypothesis am I testing, and with what kinds of controls? Following the methods I used previously in the divorce research, I selected the dreams in which the narrative features the person central to the issue at hand; in Scott's case, this is the victim, Yarmila. In most cases, I also note the type of emotion expressed within the dream. This characteristic has proved to be one of the potential elements of productive dreaming, where "productive" means regulating negative emotion within the night, and instituting changes in the self-concept that are adaptive to new circumstances. I am aware of the many pitfalls of using Scott's dreams as he notes them, but let's put these issues aside for now, while we take a dive into this unique pool of data, and see what we can find about Scott's dreams of Yarmila that offer a glimpse into how his dreaming mind addresses the act of violence he committed that ended her life and their marriage.

Selecting Dreams for Analysis

Scott was not a believer in the importance of dreams and had never paid attention to them in the past. Since he had made me a promise, though, he soldiered on. He sometimes skipped a month or more, writing in his letter to me that he was feeling lazy about making the effort to recall his dreams when he woke, to note the time of night, and to write what he could remember right away. I have now a total of 54 dreams in which Yarmila is an active character, collected over the period from September 1999 to July 2006; this means she was present in 28% of all of the dreams Scott sent to me. (The dreams used for this analysis as reported in the dream log are provided in the Appendix.)

In Scott's dreams of Yarmila, there is a detectable change over time in his image of her, the emotions he expresses in relation to her, and in his recognition that he will never have her back, even if he is released. I believe the dreams give us a number of clues about Scott's feelings toward the incident and, by extension, about his lack of intent and his remorse.

There are no dreams in which Scott is physically aggressive toward Yarmila. In only one dream, out of all 196 in the data pool, does Scott attack another person—and that was not one in which Yarmila appeared. The aggression occurred because of disparaging remarks a male character made against others. In relation to how he portrays aggression in his dreams Scott is more often escaping from others who would attack him than he is fighting back. He is frequently hiding, or seeking a safe place. I believe the dreams of Yarmila show how Scott's sleeping mind is grappling with the loss of his marriage at his own hands. One clear change that can be detected is his conception of her over time. There are three phases to this change. In the first dreams, from 1999 to 2002, she is seen as a strong, sensible, attractive, loving mate of whom he is proud. Then in the middle phase, in 2002–2004, she is the opposite: an ugly, dominant, reckless, castrating woman. In the last phase, the dreams in 2005–2006, she is going her own way and leaving Scott behind.

In Scott's earliest dreams, reported in 1999, the theme is often that he is lost or stuck, but Yarmila is always knowledgeable and supportive. In a 2000 dream, Scott is given a rifle and asked to kill a "dead" deer if it proves to be dangerous. He does not want to do this and does not have to carry this out as the deer escapes and is reunited with her family. He and Yarmila are happy to witness this. In 2001, Scott reported two dreams in which he acknowledges that he loves and misses Yarmila, but recognizes that she is gone. In a 2002 dream, he denies her death. She is pictured as loving him in a maternal manner, which "relaxes" him. In the first phase, Scott is clearly dealing with accepting her death. Two "wish fulfillment" dreams of her survival reduce his anxiety: The dead deer is in fact alive and rejoins her family, and Yarmila still actively loves Scott. These dreams function to relieve his sense of loss.

Later in 2002, in the second phase of Scott's dreams about Yarmila, he had a complicated dream in which he goes through many changes in his self-conception. He transforms from businessman, to potential religious leader, to family head, and then to a returning former prisoner. In this last role, he is given a birthday present by another woman, which creates a breach with

Yarmila. In a 2003 dream, he enjoys arranging to give Yarmila a surprise gift. That dream turns negative, as he feels responsible for changing her from a good-looking woman of whom he is proud, into a small, ugly dwarf as she "escapes" through symbols of his imprisonment (iron bars) and he is left behind. In 2004, another dream is set in prison. Again Yarmila escapes, while Scott is trapped, frozen from fear of falling. She is impatient with him. She does not understand his feeling of fear and of their real separation.

The third phase starts in a 2005 dream. Scott gives up on his idealization of Yarmila, and feels superior to her, because she is callous toward others while he is caring. In another dream later that year, Scott blames Yarmila for endangering herself and their kids, but he feels powerless to change her headstrong behavior. They are no longer equals in decision power. She has taken control. Finally, another dream in 2005 offers a bleak prospect for the future: Yarmila has no room for him on his return. On the same night, Scott dreams of walking out on Yarmila, feeling sad but right to separate from her.

In 2006, Scott dreams of a clash between them, set around the dinner hour. She changes her mind about something; he goes along but is angry about her shifting position. She is surprised to see him behave in a decisive, forceful way, but he feels good "letting my anger out." A series of 2006 dreams feature the same plot: If Scott is released, and the couple is able to eagerly rejoin, he could no longer satisfy her.

In his years of imprisonment for the violent death of his wife, Scott dreams of her frequently, and we see his emotional relationship to her shift significantly. His view of the marriage as one of equal partners, in which each is respectful of the other's strengths and weaknesses, has transmuted into one in which she dominates. He grows to accept that the relationship is no longer fulfilling. Further, Scott's emotional responses to Yarmila transform from admiration for her strength and competence to anger at her recklessness and lack of understanding of his frailty, and finally her lack of support for him. His dreams show his realization that the marriage is over emotionally. He is sad that is so and that she is the one responsible for the breach; he does everything he can to please her but nothing works.

Does Scott Consciously Acknowledge the Emotional Changes Evidenced in His Dream Reports?

I wrote to Scott asking for permission to discuss his dreams in this book, and in particular to examine them for evidence of his feelings of aggression towards Yarmila. In his response, in a letter of September 2008, he wrote that he could not recall any violent or dangerous feelings toward his wife. "I have had a few waking bouts of anger with her. In my depressed and brooding moments, I've yelled at her mentally for putting herself in harm's way that night. Why did she come outside to disturb me? Why didn't she just run away when I first attacked? She paid the price for my mismanagement of my stress and negligence in not having my sleep disorder treated. For her to take the hit is just so wrong. I still have a hard time believing it actually happened." In this waking statement, Scott projects blame for Yarmila's death onto her. "She should have known better."

What do the dreams tell us about Scott's motivation, if there was any, for murder? They do show that *post-conviction*, he experienced a gradual revision of his concept of his wife—from a partner he could count on, to someone he was unsure could accept his limitations, and then finally to someone with her own need for independence, that he can no longer trust and must abandon. This shift in his perception of their relationship, which took many years to integrate into his dreams, did not result in any act of aggression, even in the freedom of dreams.

Over the years since Yarmila's death, Scott has continued to review the relationship in his dreams, even as he accepts that his wife is gone. Most importantly, he is no longer idealizing her as the perfect partner. He now perceives her in his dreams as a more complex person, more self-involved and less supportive of him. When he and I first met while he was awaiting trial in 1998, he was still presenting her as the love of his life and ideal partner. Later, in his letter of 2008, he admits seeing her as partly responsible for her own death (although only when he is in great despair).

What has that to do with his legal and emotional culpability? Scott acknowledges his disappointment in Yarmila as a supportive mate in his dreams. Whatever his real experiences were that resulted in forming these less-than-favorable dream images, they had strong negative emotional loading. Memories of these experiences may well have been stored in Scott's long-term memory network—not just from their disagreement on the night of Yarmila's death, but over an extended time period. He may not ever have been conscious of his feelings about these experiences.

I suspect that Scott's sleepwalk that night was driven by his unconscious motivation to repair his concept of himself as a capable man, and to defend himself from anyone who would block that effort. It is entirely feasible that if Yarmila interrupted his repair work, as the police believe she did, he would have been incapable of identifying her, as he was in a brain state in which facial recognition does not function. To establish this theory as a possible defense in Scott's case, the new sleep testing protocol and spectral analysis scoring must become an accepted standard for the diagnosis of a NREM parasomnia disorder. If Scott is permitted new sleep testing, and he responds to the sleep deprivation protocol by exhibiting a behavioral arousal at the appropriate stage and timing, and if his SWS shows the signature low slow-wave activity of the sleepwalker, this could cast reasonable doubt about his guilt, and the notion that he was fully conscious on that night, as was argued by the prosecution. This strategy recently won an acquittal in another sleepwalking case, which I will present in the next chapter.

More NREM Parasomnias: Those | 6
Who Injure Themselves, Seek Food
or Sex, Explore, and Protect

In the more complex cases a sleepwalker will leave the bed
and if there are other sleepers in the house may get into bed
with them or may interact in a sexual way with other
members of the household.

—Peter Fenwick, "Sleep and sexual offending," in the journal
Medicine, Science and the Law

Violence against another person following an arousal from sleep is not the
only unusual act an adult sleepwalker may perform. Murder without
motive is but one of the family of bizarre nocturnal behaviors that are defined
as non–rapid eye movement (NREM) parasomnias. Sleep sex is apparently
much more common than sleep-related violence, and already sleepwalking has
been claimed as a defense by several people accused of inappropriate sexual
behavior. Sleep eating and, believe it or not, e-mailing while asleep may not be
crimes, but they occur surprisingly frequently. An internet site has appeared
that is devoted to sharing these experiences, and sufferers are increasingly seeking professional help. This in turn has spurred research efforts to better define
the underlying pathology of the sleepwalker, which can now be documented
whether the subject actively attempts to sleepwalk in the laboratory or not.

The new method of sleep deprivation with auditory signals, discussed in the previous chapter, is an advance for clinical diagnosis, and the new spectral analysis scoring is contributing to our understanding of the pathology involved in these disorders. The two advances bring us closer to being able to determine whether any one person has the neurological deficit that increases vulnerability to arousals from slow-wave sleep (SWS). Helpful as they are, these techniques fall short in that they do not speak to the *state of mind* during such an arousal. Was the person really unconscious? Was the attack planned, or was this a nonrational act? For this, we have to look at behavior.

As the title of this chapter indicates, the behaviors that can be undertaken during a motor arousal from SWS are many and varied. That they all belong to the same family of disorders is clear because they are all initiated soon after SWS begins, in the first or second cycle of sleep. They start with a movement arousal into some purposeful-looking but nonrational behavior. Once full waking consciousness returns, the sleeper has no memory or only very partial recall of the event. I have had patients present with all types of bizarre behaviors. I have also consulted numerous times with the families and lawyers of those who may have committed some bad act while sleepwalking, advising them on whether the act is likely to indicate a sleep disorder diagnosis or is more likely to be due to some other real or (in some cases) fictitious complaint.

Sleepwalkers are of great interest to me because what they do in their half-awake/half-asleep mind state allows us to witness directly the psychology driving their behavior. Presently, our knowledge of what goes on in the mind during REM sleep is based on the sleepers' reports of what they remember of their dreams. In the NREM parasomnias, we can judge the behavior for ourselves and at least speculate about it, without the potentially confounding influence of the sleeper's own account of what was going on. In the case of understanding dreams, sleep researchers are twice removed from the original data.

Self-injury Cases

Some sleepwalkers injure not others but themselves. I have had patients who jumped out of their bedroom windows, and others who thrust an arm through a glass door or window. All were young men and none were suicidal, but all did extensive damage to themselves without any apparent motive or memory. This had the benefit of bringing them in to be diagnosed and treated, rather than going to jail.

Patients with sleep disorders often try to apply a logical explanation to what is essentially irrational behavior. One young man who jumped out his window defended his act by telling me that he may have fallen out unintentionally while trying to open the window wider. He explained that it was a hot summer night and that he was sleeping without pajamas—in fact, in nothing at all. His window was open part way with a small sliding screen at the opening. He remembered checking the time on his bedside digital clock just before he fell asleep. It was 12:05 A.M. He had no memory of what happened, next. He "awoke" on the pavement two stories below his window. People were calling out from their windows above, "Are you all right?" He was not. He felt something warm and wet beneath him. He was lying in a pool of his own blood. Nonetheless, he got up and walked to his second floor apartment door, which was locked. As he had no key, he rang the doorbell of the apartment across the hall. That tenant took one look and called 911; the operator logged the call at 12:17 A.M. Clearly, he had been in his first NREM sleep of the night when the incident occurred. He had extensive injuries, including a punctured lung and spleen, broken ribs, and severe damage to both legs. He spent 6 months in rehab and then came to our sleep center.

Another young man, who went out the window of his college dorm room in his sleep, was not as badly hurt; however, once he recovered, university officials were loath to take responsibility for having him live on campus. The student was determined to finish his degree program. We put him on the standard pharmaceutical treatment for this disorder (a small dose of the drug clonazepam at bedtime). He took a quarter off to live at home under the watchful eye of his mother, to be sure there would be no further incidents. There were none, and he returned to finish his degree, living in an off-campus apartment.

Such events are not only potentially life-threatening but, if patients survive, the fallout can be mind-changing and potentially career-changing. One patient came in after thrusting his arm through his bedroom window. The left arm was bandaged from shoulder to palm. He had torn nerves as well as muscles and tendons. A violinist, he was afraid that he would have to give up music, but he mended well.

Another young man thrust his arm through a pane of glass on his sleepwalking way out the door. Later, he remembered something that had happened the day before that might have shed some light on what was on his mind, and why this happened. He and a friend were walking on a city street when a gang of tough-looking kids surrounded them. He was afraid they would be attacked. The gang demanded their money. The young man calculated his odds and decided discretion was the better part of valor; he handed over his wallet. His friend did not, and the gang fled with only my patient's money and I.D. He felt humiliated in the eyes of his friend for having given in. He did not want anyone else to know, and he did not tell his parents. The incident was on his mind as he fell asleep that night. Shame and a loss of esteem in the eyes of others is a common prelude to sleep-related violence in many NREM parasomnia patients.

All of these young men had been sleeping alone when their episodes occurred. Would having a partner in the bed have been safer for them? Not really. A case in point: A young married man, while sleeping, flung an arm, striking his wife in the face. She interpreted it as an intended punch. She had been subject to this often enough to go to bed armed. She retaliated by dousing him with the glass of water she kept on her bedside table. He then jumped out of bed, still not fully conscious. To her, he looked "scary," so she scampered to escape. He threw scissors at her, barely missing her head, but they were thrown with such force that one blade stuck in the wall. She fled in her nightie to the garage, attempting to drive out of harm's way. He followed and in bare feet kicked at the garage door hard enough to break it. His foot took a beating too; this is what woke him, ending the episode (and the marriage).

A similar marriage-ending episode was part of the history a new patient reported when he came to my office for his first appointment. His first wife had ended their marriage after waking on several occasions to find his hands around her throat. He remarried, only for his second wife to have the same experience. By that time, the knowledge that this might be a treatable sleep disorder had brought him in to ask for help. He has been able to control his sleep disorder for the past 6 years using the standard drug treatment.

Sleep Eating

Unlike those who are violent, who are predominantly male, the sleep eaters are more likely to be evenly distributed across both genders. They get up, go to the kitchen, and prepare and eat foods. The problem is what they eat—foods that they would not find palatable if they were fully conscious. For instance, one patient ate a box of cookie mix directly out of the package. Some take the food back to bed with them and wake in the morning to find the remains of a meal littering their sheets. Others make for the outdoors and go shopping, often for foods they do not usually hanker for. Commonly, sleep eaters will have an episode of sleep eating when they are not spending the night in their own beds. "I was visiting my daughter and son-in-law," one man told me, when he got up and went to the kitchen and started a fry-up of all sorts of incompatible items from the refrigerator. Luckily, the smoke this produced set off an alarm, which brought the son-in-law downstairs to investigate. He then led the sleepwalking chef back to bed.

A nephew of mine, while visiting his uncle in another city, took an Ambien to help him sleep. He was found fast asleep with his head on the kitchen table while a large pot of vinegar bubbled on the stove. Sliced bananas were simmering in it. He had not been a sleepwalker prior to this episode, but apparently the strange environment had made him more alert, and the Ambien was the immediate trigger for his sleepwalk and cooking. Luckily, he did not try to eat what he was preparing.

One patient of ours was a young and attractive woman, newly married, who was trying hard to keep her weight down by restricting her food intake during the day. She would sleepwalk to the kitchen every night, and indiscriminately eat whatever was available. She had no recall of these episodes and was thoroughly committed to getting control of this, as her nightly walks were regularly defeating her waking weight maintenance program. We worked on having her gratify her hunger during the day instead. That did not stop her night eating. Next, I thought to prescribe something to help her sleep through the first SWS period and get safely into REM. She balked at taking a sleeping pill, so I tried L-tryptophan for her (it was then still available over-the-counter in this country). She called and reported with great enthusiasm that she was cured: "It's working. I am feeling so full, and I don't get up to eat any more." I might have fooled myself into thinking that this was a success case, except for her follow-up report. Six months after she declared herself "cured," she told me that she was still sleeping through the night, but gaining weight. She added, somewhat sheepishly, that her feeling of fullness turned out to be a result of her then-unsuspected pregnancy.

Sleep Sex

Sleep sex has become something of a darling of the internet. Many who are affected blog about the sexual exploits they have experienced with a sleeping partner. Some partners of these sexually active bedmates find the behavior annoying, while others enjoy it, saying it is better than their usual waking love-making experience. Sleep sex is often described as "rougher" than regular intercourse, or, somewhat unsettlingly, more like rape. I was slow to catch on that this was another NREM parasomnia when a patient arrived with his wife following an arrest for indecent exposure. She had observed that he often masturbated shortly after sleep onset. At first, she assumed that his sleepwalking was just a bathroom trip. Instead, he would stand with his back to the bedroom door frame and masturbate. The incident that got him into legal trouble and caused him to come to the Sleep Center for help occurred as he waited in his car to pick her up from work. He fell asleep while waiting and, as he was parked in a restricted area, a policeman looked into the driver's window to warn him to move on. Instead, he was arrested.

At that time, there were no such cases in our diagnostic manual. However, an article had appeared in the *Singapore Medical Journal* in 1986, entitled "Masturbation during sleep—a somnambulistic variant?" There it was, identified in print. Since then, numerous journal articles have been published identifying sleep sex as another NREM parasomnia. In most of the cases that involved an arrest, the charges were brought not by a bed partner but rather by an adult stranger or on behalf of a child. In these cases, the initial part of the episode involves a sleepwalk to another bedroom, to the bedroom of a neighbor across the street, or even to a distant location. Some of these cases involve only a touch, which awakens and frightens the sleeper, who screams; help comes, and so do the police. Has the sleepwalker become a sex predator? Is this a different disorder, or a variant of sleepwalking?

One patient reported that he had lain down on top of a child who was spending the night at his house in a sleeping bag on his living room floor. He did not try to get into the bag—he just fell asleep there, frightening the child. Another sleepwalker went somewhat further; the man fondled one of his own sleeping children and spent time in a court-mandated counseling program. He was forbidden from returning to live with his family for a year. This man was not my patient, but he e-mailed me about his case, and I urged him to seek the medication (clonazepam) that we have found works best in these cases. He is now back living with his family, and he sent me a photo of them all together. I noted that, like many other adult sleepwalkers, he was a big man, both tall and heavy.

The Good Neighbor Case

The Good Neighbor was such a stable, big, all-around decent guy that he was asked by those who lived on either side of him to check on their homes when they were away. One long holiday weekend when both sets of neighbors were out of town, he was put in charge. He had been under a good deal of stress, as his wife had had a troubled pregnancy and had required bed rest in her last trimester. She had just delivered and was staying, along with their two other small children, at her mother's house in a neighboring town. The Good Neighbor had to work, so he was at home alone. He remembered drinking a good deal of coffee on the morning before the incident, followed by diet cola drinks through-out a busy day packed with activities he needed to keep on schedule. His responsibilities continued into the evening, and he kept up his diet cola con-sumption. When his work was done, he checked the neighbors' houses and then went to sleep.

What happened next is rather muddled, but the scenario the police put together is that he got up shortly after 1:00 A.M. with a sense of urgency, believed he "saw" lights on in the house across the street, and felt he had to check it out. He did not know that neighbor and had not been asked to look after that house. Nonetheless, he crossed the street and entered the unlocked front door (he lived in a small town where this was not unusual). He went into the master bedroom, where the family's teenage daughter was sleeping with her boyfriend. He stood over the bed and, as she alleged later, "touched or stroked" her thigh. She woke, screaming at him to get out. In his confused state, he blundered into the kitchen. The young lady then led him to the front door and watched as he returned home where he slept through the rest of the night. Next morning, the girl's mother returned home and was told the story of an intruder. She called the police, who arrested our Good Neighbor. He was very surprised, thinking that as soon as he explained his sleepwalking problem he could apologize and be permitted to go home. He had a long history of sleepwalking, well known to his family and friends.

The trouble did not go away. The Good Neighbor was charged with home invasion, which is a felony. He was also charged with intent to commit a sexual assault. He retained a good lawyer and was advised to contact a sleep expert, which is when I entered the picture. I took his history, scored his overnight sleep study, and testified for him when his case came to trial. He was a devoted husband and father, respected by those he worked with, but he waited for an uncomfortable 2 years for his day in court.

Perhaps the most interesting aspect of this case involves the amount of caf-feine the Good Neighbor had ingested throughout the day before the incident. Caffeine not only helps to keep people awake during the day, it also lightens the first cycle of sleep, making arousals more frequent (just as Ambien does, some-what paradoxically). As I mentioned earlier, I believe caffeine may have played a role in the Falater case, too. Scott was taking caffeine tablets to stay focused at work and to counteract the sleepiness caused by his troubled nights.

The Good Neighbor's sleep study was scored using both the traditional scor-ing and the newer spectral analysis scoring, which is a finer-grained analysis of brain waves, as it counts the number of waves that fall within the delta range in each sleep cycle of the night. The study revealed that his sleep had significantly low delta activity in the first sleep cycle, characteristic of sleepwalkers who are easily aroused from slow wave sleep (SWS). This supported his sleepwalking defense against the home invasion charge. I felt that the sleep sex charge was less than credible, as the teenager did not mention the physical contact to her boyfriend, did not call 911, and did not seem to fear the Good Neighbor as she led him to the front door. The jury agreed, and he was acquitted on all charges.

The sleep sex disorder occurs in both genders, although it seems more common in males than in females at about a 3:2 ratio. These data have not yet been confirmed, as they are based on an unscientific sample survey posted on a website. What links sleep sex to other NREM parasomnias is the difficulty of awakening fully; sleepwalkers remain in an in-between partial wake state, only gradually becoming fully conscious. Their behavior seems somehow "primitive" (seeking satisfaction of the biological drive for sexual gratification). They have no memory of what took place, and subsequently feel a good deal of embarrassment and shame. They also frequently have a history of childhood sleepwalking or sleep terrors, or they have a family member who does. These characteristics make for a strong case that sleep sex is a true sleep disorder of the NREM parasomnia type.

We have seen a variety of semi-sleep/semi-wake behaviors—involving aggression, hunger, and sex. All of these are strong, basic drives that we all share. The sleepwalkers' behavior appears to express the need to satisfy one or more of these drives, seeming to erupt in an unsocialized form out of deep sleep. Sleep sex behaviors are now appearing more frequently as legal cases in which the sleepwalker faces a jury that must decide guilt or innocence. Citizens who become jurors need help in understanding how best to judge the defendant's responsibility in these cases. These are not easy decisions to make, and are far more complex than are the basic facts of the case. Juries and judges must go beyond deciding whether a defendant did or did not lie down next to or on top of a sleeping child. An equally important question is, in what frame of mind was the defendant when this inappropriate behavior was performed?

REM Sleep Erections

It has long been known that REM sleep is accompanied by a penile erection cycle in males and sexual arousal in females, indicated by an increase in vaginal blood flow. This physiological arousal is not associated with sexual content in dreams; instead, it happens regularly along with any dream story, even the most mundane. The only exception is an anxiety dream, which will lead to a dip in an ongoing erection in men. The erection cycle usually recovers and continues unless an awakening takes place. Sleep sex behavior, however, does not appear to be related to this normal cycle of penile tumescence in REM sleep. I entertained the idea that erections during sleep might be the mechanism behind sleep sex behavior because, normally, the erection begins just prior to the signs of REM sleep—when the brain waves change to those of low amplitude with rapid frequency, just before the drop of muscle tone at the chin that follows, and then, last, the rapid eye movements that confirm this is the beginning of a REM sleep episode. The erection lasts throughout the REM period, with detumescence not occurring until after there is a change back to NREM sleep. It seemed possible that sleep sex behavior might be a transitional error stimulated by the onset of a normal pre-REM erection. This hypothesis has neither been proven nor thrown out. I believe the reason is that sleep labs are no longer asked to do these erection evaluations to aid in the diagnosis and treatment of impotence. When Viagra came along, erectile-dysfunction patients were no longer referred for sleep studies, as their problem could be addressed easily with a prescription. Sleep labs have not yet considered the use of penile strain gauges for sleep sex evaluations. These might offer a clearer picture of where in sleep the internal stimulus for sleep sex behavior originates.

If sleep sex behaviors are part of the physiological sexual arousal cycle that occurs just prior to REM, one fact that might support this notion is that compulsive masturbation does not seem to be as closely related to the first SWS period of the night as are other NREM parasomnias. In other words, while other NREM parasomnias occur almost exclusively during the first deep sleep, sleep-related masturbation and initiation of sexual activity with a bed partner may follow a different time course; bed partners report this happens at various times throughout the night, as does REM sleep.

When I have a clinical hunch such as this one, I find it is best to go back to patients and ask more questions in the hopes that I may find important new details. I had the opportunity to do this with a particularly memorable case of compulsive masturbatory sleep sex. A man and his wife came to the Sleep Center together, explaining that he had developed a new sleep behavior that was most troublesome to her ability to sleep. He was masturbating in bed several times every night. His movements woke her each time, and she wanted her sleep integrity respected. They had been married for 15 years, had children and had, and continued to have, a good sex life. Having intercourse before sleep did not deter his self-stimulation later in the night. This being a new behavior, the couple was able to relate the timing of its onset to a major emotionally disturbing event: The husband had failed to get an anticipated job promotion. He had been passed over in favor of another candidate. He was very disappointed and felt that he had been treated unfairly. Like the teenager who gave up his wallet without a fight, this man felt ashamed of his passivity in not challenging the decision—in short, he felt symbolically castrated. So strong was the emotional component to his self-soothing sleep sex behavior that I suggested he be treated with hypnotherapy instead of pharmacotherapy. Hypnosis works quickly, and as the technique for self-hypnosis is mastered, it has the added advantage of restoring the patient's sense of self-control. That would take care of his sleep symptom and restore her sleep; but I also recommended psychotherapy, as the patient needed to develop better methods of coping with authority. He has been taught self-hypnosis to control the troublesome behavior, and is now working with a psychotherapist on repairing his self-esteem, revising his self-concept, and improving interpersonal skills.

The Explorers

Like other NREM parasomnia patients, those I refer to as "explorers" get up out of their first SWS and take off. Some drive, some climb, some run. Usually nothing much happens unless they crash their cars, as happened to a certain congressman at 2 A.M.—an event that made national news. The police records indicate that when they arrived at the scene, the man was in a confused mental state, telling them he was on his way to cast his vote. He had taken Ambien, which, as I have noted, does help sleep continuity, but also has the effect of lightening SWS. (Ambien is now labeled with a warning that it might precipitate sleepwalking, driving, and eating.)

A more typical sleep explorer was a woman who also got into her car and crashed into a fire hydrant near her home. She left the car, walked home, and went back to sleep. When the police came the next morning to inquire why she had not reported her accident, she could not answer them because she had no memory of what had occurred. She could not report where she was going or why. The police were not charmed. She was ticketed for a DUI (driving under the influence). She paid a fine but protested that this accident was not alcohol-related. She wanted her record cleared. This cost her a good deal in legal fees but eventually she won her case. Happily, no one was hurt.

Another sleep explorer was not so fortunate. He was grieving the death of his son and not sleeping well at night. On one occasion, he took both an Ambien and a tumbler of alcohol in order to get a good night's sleep. What he was aware of next was awakening and wondering why the police were pulling him out of his bed. A moment later he realized that he was actually being pulled out of his car, still parked in his driveway. He was sound asleep, the Ambien and alcohol having caused him to arouse, without awareness of what he was doing, and get into his car. He could not say where he planned to go. He was charged with a DUI even though he never got the car started. This time, the charges stuck.

A 15-year-old girl got up from sleep and climbed to the end of a construction crane, 130 feet above ground level, where she curled up and fell asleep. Someone spotted her and took a photograph, which appeared in the *London Daily Mail*. Her mother had alerted the emergency services that her daughter was missing and that she was a sleepwalker. She was quickly found, but officials were afraid to approach her for fear of startling her in her precarious position. Knowing that the girl's cell phone was in her backpack, her mother gave the rescuers the number. They called, she woke, and they brought her down safely.

A news story out of Iowa City reported on another explorer, a marathon runner and college student with a sleepwalking history. He was spotted by several drivers running in his underwear shorts down an interstate highway at 1 A.M. Before the state police could track him down he had been hit by a car and did not survive.

These sleepers are not aggressive, hungry, or sexually inappropriate. Instead they are simply driven by an impulse to be out and about, exploring when they should be fast asleep. We assume that the desire to explore is part of the bundle of basic drives that continue to motivate humans in various ways. In these instances of sleepwalking, this archival drive appears to break through the restraints of deep sleep in those who have a genetic flaw in the system that, for most of us, inhibits motor activity during SWS.

The Protectors

This group of sleepers displays a unique pattern of behavior during NREM parasomnia episodes. Earlier I related the historical case of a woman who threw her baby out a window, believing her house was on fire. In terms of her misperception of the situation, she was acting as a protector. One of my own patients dragged his wife out of bed thinking the mattress was on fire. He also thought he was protecting her; she thought otherwise.

The first patient I ever saw with this complaint was a big, good-looking young man who had recently moved into a loft apartment converted from a defunct factory. He lived there alone. One night, he told me, he found himself at the window pulling the wainscoting off the frame, convinced that his brother and sister-in-law were buried within. He pulled off a good deal of wood with his bare hands before waking in confusion. And this was not his only adventure in this new abode. On another night, he found himself lifting his king-sized water bed to free his nephew, who he believed was stuck underneath. Both of these acts required a lot of strength and effort and, while misguided, were well intentioned.

These cases make interesting stories but beyond that are instructive as we begin to see some psychological sense in apparently nonsensical behaviors. This is important to our understanding of the motivations ongoing during the sleep with which we begin the night.

Sleep Behavior in the Young

Before opening my first sleep lab in 1963, I had the chance to observe the work being done by Anthony Kales in his University of California, Los Angeles lab. I was teaching there for a summer session. Kales, a psychiatrist, was studying sleepwalking children, and he allowed me to watch how he and his team had overcome the problem of monitors limiting the sleepwalkers' movements while hooked up to the many electrodes needed to record their sleep. In that laboratory, a very long cable was held by the technician, almost like a leash. The sleepwalking child was followed as he or she roamed around the lab—all while still being recorded. This allowed them to examine the state of the child's brain waves during the walk.

Were these walkers awake or asleep? They were not exclusively in either state, but in a mixture of both. When the children first got up from bed, they were clearly still producing the high-amplitude slow waves of delta sleep. Shortly after they arose, the brain waves became a mixture of theta, alpha, and beta rhythms, and then, finally, a fully awake state was exhibited. During their walks, the children had normal reflex responses—a knee jerk to a light hammer tap, withdrawal from a pin prick. Kales summed up his experience by writing that these children "appear to have impaired ability to incorporate all sensory input into cortical awareness or at least to act on it appropriately. . . . We cannot say that somnambulists are asleep during the incidents, although they certainly begin during slow wave sleep. On the other hand we cannot call this an awake state. It is a distinctive state of somnambulism."

As noted earlier, studies show that the prevalence of sleepwalking and sleep terrors is much higher in children than in adults. Although estimates vary, a ballpark figure of 20% of children between the ages of 3 and 12 will have NREM arousals from their early delta sleep. This figure is based on a study of both children and adults who had arousals associated with sleepwalking, sleep terrors with sleep talking, and nocturnal enuresis (bed wetting after the age of 5).

If we also include children who have the occasional confusional arousal, the percentage climbs to 40%–50%. Of these, it is estimated that 25% will continue to have a chronic sleepwalking problem that persists into adulthood. Sleepwalkers were first studied extensively in France and then Canada in the early 1960s, culminating in a landmark 1968 article in the journal *Science* by Roger Broughton, a neurologist. He defined these NREM events as a group of related "disorders of arousal" from SWS. He also showed that these episodes were followed by a longer confusional state after a delta sleep arousal than usually follows a REM sleep arousal.

To instigate sleepwalking in the laboratory in his young patients Broughton stood them up while they were in their first long delta sleep period. Once on their feet, away they would go. They still had the muscle tone that allowed them to ambulate before REM left them profoundly relaxed. Another trick Broughton used was to load the children with fluids before bedtime—sometimes the pressure of a full bladder is enough to start a walk, but he also got some wet beds. Nocturnal enuresis is part of the history we look for in sleepwalkers of all ages because it indicates a difficulty with coming to full wakefulness from deep sleep in time to make it to the proper place to urinate. Lots of stories in the sleep literature report patients urinating in a closet, a waste basket, on a couch—even standing on a grand piano. Broughton showed that his enuretics had more bladder contractions and higher bladder pressure throughout all their sleep than did nonenuretic children.

With great imagination, Broughton experimented with various new ways to trigger NREM parasomnia behavior. He used sounds, called the children's names, positioned them on their feet, filled their bladders. He found lifting them to the floor worked best for the little ones who had a history of sleepwalking, and that this did not produce walking in those without this history. Too bad this was not appropriate for adults, especially the big ones. This early experience of the 1960s has been revisited by a research group working in Montreal under the direction of Jacques Montplaisir. Montplaisir and his colleagues are responsible for both of the new methods for diagnosing sleepwalking in the laboratory.

NREM Parasomnias: Common Features

The term "overlap disorder" describes those patients who appear to have more than one of these sleep-related behaviors on different nights, or even during the same night. This overlap supports the notion that these NREM parasomnias are related, and may originate from the same set of risk factors. For example,

I believe that Scott Falater's attack on his wife started as a benign sleepwalking episode, and that it did not turn violent until she interrupted his intended "good deed." At that point Scott, behaved in an attack–defense mode of behavior resembling that of a child who beats the person attempting to restrain him during a sleep terror event. The difference in Scott's case is that he did not exhibit sleep terror symptoms when he first arose from bed. He did not let loose the signature scream, or exhibit other signs of panic behavior. His attack on his wife occurred some time after he first arose, when his sleepwalking episode was interrupted. This would suggest that, on occasion, sleep-related violence can be an overlap disorder combining aspects of sleepwalking and sleep terrors in the same event.

I have noted that in many of these cases an ongoing emotional issue has been disruptive to sleep for some period of time before the sleepwalking event occurs. In the divorce dream studies, some of the volunteers did and some did not manage to successfully reduce negative emotions in their dreams. In NREM parasomnia cases, sleepers never achieve REM before they take action. As a result, the negative emotions have not been down-regulated, and this drives the behavior that is enacted in sleepwalking episodes. I illustrated this point in detail in discussing Scott's case, and in describing the compulsive sleep masturbator who was passed over for promotion. Ken Parks' murder of his mother-in-law was preceded by months of worry about his compulsive gambling and consequent debts. His story was so compelling that it became the basis of a made-for-TV movie. Ken was another apparently well-intended man who, when unable to take rational action toward solving his financial dilemma, and unable to sleep because of worry, had a benign sleepwalking episode that, in his nonrational state, led to his carrying out a promise to his wife to visit his in-laws. He, too, was interrupted, and then attacked. These cases all implicate ongoing anxiety, caused by a perceived serious threat to the individual's self-system, leading to a chronic state of sleep deprivation that undermines the positive functions of sleep.

Unusual strength and/or endurance is another characteristic that many NREM parasomnia cases share. Scott stabbed his wife 44 times; Ken beat his father-in-law into unconsciousness before repeatedly stabbing his mother-in-law. The man who threw scissors at his wife did so with such force that they stuck in the wall and hung there. A protector lifted his water bed. We know that people can perform unusual feats of strength under extreme emergency circumstances while wide awake. In wartime, men have been known to carry the body of an injured buddy for miles while under fire. This takes the mobilization of stress hormones to provide the extra energy required to perform these acts. What is the emergency in NREM parasomnia cases? Unfortunately, the threat is not real (though the consequences are); instead, the threat is psychological in nature—the breakdown of the sleepwalker's positive self-image. In NREM parasomnias, a psychological crisis seems to mobilize unusual physical strength.

Several of the men in these cases I described were big, tall, and young. Ken stood 6 feet 5 inches tall; his mother-in-law had nicknamed him "the gentle giant." The man who attempted to strangle his wife was over 6 feet; so too were the Good Neighbor and the man who was charged with molesting one of his own children. How could physical size have anything to do with sleepwalking episodes? Remember that the largest peak of human growth hormone is released in the first SWS cycle of the night. Not all NREM parasomnia patients are super-sized, but enough of them are large people to raise a question about the role of hormones in the development of disordered sleep. And how does gender contribute to an individual's vulnerability to these disorders, since there is such a predominance of males who are implicated in adult sleep-related violence cases? Studies have shown that violent sleepwalkers, both men and women, have high testosterone levels. Another clue.

What other characteristics do these people share? How about what they do while sleepwalking? Psychologists by training look for meaning in behavior, and these patients all do things that are apparently *very unlike* them in their conscious waking lives. They are often exceptionally good people who, while having an episode, behave very badly. They strike out against loved ones, do damage to their own property, injure themselves, they eat peculiar noxious foods, are sexually unrestrained, and engage in dangerous explorations. These are all strong drives that we are taught to curb as we are socialized according to the rules of our culture. Are sleepwalkers characteristically over-controlling of basic drives, lacking the flexibility of response when some new adaptation is required? I would vote "yes" to this description for those I know. Furthermore, this dogged self-control, which may reach obsessive–compulsive proportions, has also been pointed out as a personality characteristic of sleepwalkers in the older legal literature.

What about the timing of these behaviors—any similarities there? I have repeatedly pointed out that sleepwalkers arise from the deep sleep that occurs at the beginning of the night, in either the first or the second sleep cycle. These behaviors do not originate in REM, nor do they happen toward morning. This places them within the first third of the night's sleep, in delta sleep. These behaviors are episodic—not occurring every night. This is an important point for psychologists because it indicates variability, which offers the opportunity to look into why the behavior happened on one night and not on others. Apparently something besides a genetic predisposition and sleep deprivation is needed to push the brain to produce more SWS, eventually causing an abnormal sleep arousal.

A NREM parasomnia event is also more likely to occur when the sleeper is sleeping in a strange location, or in a new or unfamiliar bed. This makes for a more alert sleep state, a lighter sleep. The sleeper's safety "cues"—the feel of the mattress, weight of the blankets, odors in the air, and light or darkness of the room—are different from those of their usual environment. They are therefore more easily aroused.

Why? Why cannot these individuals sleep through to REM? Why do they instead rise, sleepwalk, explore, protect, or seek food or sexual release? I have outlined what I see as the elements common to all of the cases discussed in this chapter: sleep deprivation, chronic stress, perhaps use or abuse of a sleep aid or other substance that acts contrary to the sleep-deprivation deepening effect, a genetic abnormality that fails to inhibit motor activity during SWS, and so on. It appears that, in many cases, the need to repair one's self-esteem is at the basis of what motivates some sleepwalking behavior. This does not, however, account for all NREM parasomnias. I will return to this issue in Chapter 10 when I present my own theoretical model for the sleeping mind.

Sleepwalking and State of Mind in the Courtroom

> In 1686, [Sir Peter Lely] was indicted at the Old Bailey, for
> shooting one of the guards, and his horse to boot. He
> pleaded somnambulism, and was acquitted on producing
> nearly fifty witnesses, to prove the extraordinary things he
> did in his sleep.
>
> —Robert Macnish, *The Philosophy of Sleep*

The rise in public awareness of sleep disorders, as well as the media frenzy surrounding cases like Scott Falater's and Ken Parks', has been something of a mixed blessing for those of us in the field. It has led to a sharp increase in patients applying for help, to the extent that the number of patients far exceeds the availability of trained personnel and properly equipped and staffed laboratories. This was pointed out in the report published in 2006 by the Institute of Medicine referred to previously. That book, *Sleep Disorders and Sleep Deprivation*, has a subtitle *An Unmet Public Health Problem* that says it all. There is a clear need to catch up to this demand by training more physicians and clinical psychologists to diagnose and treat patients using evidenced-based, high-quality care.

On top of this, more and more frequently sleep clinicians are being asked to serve as expert witnesses when a sleep disorder gets someone into trouble with the law. Lawyers, family members, friends, and even defendants themselves need help understanding (and using as a legitimate defense in court) the nature of potentially dangerous sleep disorders. We have seen that there are many ways in which a non–rapid eye movement (NREM) parasomnia can result in criminal charges. These range from driving under the influence (DUI), to breaking and entering with intent to commit a felony, sexual misconduct, indecent exposure, assault, and so on, up to and including homicide.

Sleep scientists and sleep clinicians have been reluctant to enter these uncharted waters. The questions they are asked on the witness stand are not those they are accustomed to answering. For instance, the basic question, "What was the defendant's state of mind while committing this crime?" is unanswerable, and this single question prevents many experts from agreeing to testify under oath. Scientists can weigh in on the likelihood of whether a given person is a sleepwalker, but not what that person was thinking or feeling during an episode (or even if a sleepwalking episode has definitely taken place on that occasion). If a man is able to carry out a complex motor act, like driving a car for a long distance while obeying traffic signals, as Ken Parks did, or changing clothes and working to repair the motor on a pool pump, as Scott Falater did, and then displays behaviors that show a lack of rational judgment about when and what they are doing, how are we to judge his state of mind on that specific night, and thus his degree of legal responsibility—especially if he returned to normal functioning once he became fully awake?

For the most part, the guiding principle in the legal arena is what is known as *mens rea*—was there a culpable state of mind at the time? Did the person know the behavior constituted a crime? This concept is different from an insanity plea, which the American Law Institute defines as: "A defendant is not criminally responsible if, as a result of a mental disease or defect, he lacks substantial capacity to either appreciate the criminality of his conduct or to conform his conduct to the requirements of the law." Both of these principles require conscious awareness that the act is wrongful if defendants are to be judged responsible. This puts sleep experts on the spot to swear, with a reasonable degree of certainty, that the acts with which defendants are charged were carried out while their minds were not capable of appreciating that what they were doing constituted a criminal act. As sleepwalking is an episodic behavior, not occurring every night, and in some sleepwalkers occurring only rarely, it is understandably difficult for some experts to testify that an act they have not personally witnessed was likely carried out during a time in which the defendant was in an impaired state of mind.

Compounding this difficulty, and unknown to many who look for help at sleep disorder centers, is the fact that many of the professionals who now staff these centers came to this specialtiy after training in pulmonary medicine—not psychiatry or psychology. They are not likely to have enough experience with sleep disorders, other than those of breathing disorders, to be helpful. Primary care physicians refer patients to a sleep center if they present with symptoms of excessive daytime sleepiness, obesity, hypertension, and a history of raucous snoring, because they are aware of the need to evaluate these patients for obstructive sleep apnea (OSA). This cluster of symptoms has become so familiar as an indicator of a prevalent sleep disorder that many pulmonary specialists have transitioned into the field of sleep medicine as a growth area for medical practice. Physicians are required to complete an additional year of training in an accredited sleep disorder service before taking the board examination that qualifies them to evaluate and treat sleep patients. Rarely will they see enough patients with sleepwalking during that training year to be able to assess the credibility of someone who has been charged with wrongdoing. They are not qualified to testify as expert witnesses in sleepwalking cases unless the case involves an overlap of sleepwalking and OSA.

Sleepwalking and Sleep Apnea

Remember that a period of sleep deprivation before a NREM parasomnia event is frequently mentioned in the case histories of sleepwalkers. Disrupted sleep is also a feature of OSA. When there is a loss of tone in the muscles that hold the upper airway open during sleep and the regular breathing rhythm is thus halted for at least 10 seconds, the level of oxygen carried in the bloodstream drops. This causes the patient to arouse and take a gasping breath. In severe cases, these arousals disrupt sleep up to 60 or more times per hour of sleep. Most of these occur in REM sleep, when the loss of muscle tone is dramatic, but they are also common in NREM sleep when patients are overweight, sleep on their backs, and have upper airways crowded with fatty deposits or swollen from efforts to breathe through narrow openings. If such a person also has a genetic predisposition for sleepwalking, he or she may experience a breathing arousal that turns into a motor behavior in a confusional state. In other words, such a person may have two diagnoses—a double whammy. In these instances, sleep apnea may be a trigger for a NREM parasomnia episode.

One such man contacted me by letter in April 1997, asking for help after having been convicted of first-degree murder in the shooting of his wife. He had been sentenced to life without parole in 1994, and was seeking a retrial in the hopes of overturning that conviction. This was an especially interesting case, as the man had been hospitalized for heart failure in February 1994, 2 months after the shooting but before his case came to trial. He was diagnosed then with severe sleep apnea, and an emergency tracheostomy was performed to bypass his obstructed upper airway.

The physician who took care of him during that hospitalization, a pulmonologist, performed two follow-up sleep tests in July 1994. In the first test, the tracheostomy was closed to see if the 6-month interval of breathing through the surgical opening had reduced the swelling of the patient's upper airway, perhaps improving his breathing disorder. This test proved the patient still had severe OSA. The count of "respiratory events" that night was 448, or 124 per hour of sleep, with the blood oxygen level dropping to as low as 63%. The patient's sleep was fragmented by 164 arousals, with 27 awakenings lasting over 1 minute each. During the second sleep test, the tracheostomy remained closed, and the patient was given the standard treatment for severe OSA, called nasal continuous positive airway pressure (CPAP). He slept with a mask into which 4 liters of oxygen were administered, and his throat was forced to remain open with pressurized room air delivered through tubing from bedside equipment that controlled the amount of pressure. This improved the patient's ability to sleep and breathe, although the report showed that higher pressure would be needed to ensure better control of his respiration in future.

The pulmonologist testified at the murder trial about the patient's diagnosed OSA, saying that this was one of the most severe cases he had seen. The patient was so profoundly sleepy during the day that he frequently fell asleep while driving and while at work. He fit the profile of an OSA patient not only because of his sleep tests and daytime sleepiness, but also because he was a big man—well over 300 pounds. Like Rechtschaffen's sleep-deprived rats described in Chapter 3, the patient had the bad temper of a profoundly sleep-deprived person.

What about the evidence of NREM parasomnias in this case? I responded to the man's letter and asked him whether he had a history of sleepwalking incidents. He replied that his wife had told him of his "fighting with people in his sleep, using foul language, and tearing the bed covers off. She had shown me bruises on her arms and legs and told me it was from me kicking her at night in the bed." At the trial, the pulmonologist/sleep expert testified as to the nature of the patient's history: "His father had already reported sleepwalking and lots of talking and behaviors. At that time, and this was October prior to the incident, the question of sleep disorders was raised by his physician." Later, when asked about sleep-related violence, this expert responded "there is no question about that. No question by anybody's review that at this time he had severe sleep fragmentation and sleep drunkenness." (Sleep drunkenness is a term used for the prolonged mental confusion following an arousal, especially arousals from delta, or slow-wave, sleep). He went on in his testimony to state that "We know when he was jailed after the incident that he actually had an accident where he dreamed he was being attacked and threw himself out of bed and hit the bars." This could have been an apnea arousal, but whether it was from REM or NREM sleep remains unknown.

In sum, the defense presented the case as a man suffering from severe OSA, with a history of daytime sleepiness, of about ten years' duration. The defendant had sought help from his family physician because he was having increasing trouble remaining vigilant while driving and working. That doctor believed he should be tested for sleep apnea, but the patient had decided to put this off until after the Christmas holidays. His lawyer noted that the defendant had no police record, and that the shooting of his wife, for which he claimed to have no memory, was accidental. The incident had occurred approximately 45 minutes after the defendant's onset to sleep. The gun was kept between the headboard and the mattress of their queen-sized waterbed. It was purchased after two incidents of prowlers sighted at their mobile home. It was the sound of the shot that woke the defendant fully, and when he could not rouse his wife he called 911. The call was made at approximately 2:15 A.M.

The coroner testified in support of this being an accidental shooting on the basis of the angle of the shot and the position of the weapon. In the transcript he states, "the way it was fired. . . . It wasn't aimed." ("Why do you say that?") The coroner answered "Because it was flat on the bed." A woman who read a news story about the case offered to testify that she too kept a gun under her pillow and had shot it once during sleep, thinking she was being attacked by two men trying to kill her. She had a diagnosed sleep disorder and described her state as "confused and disoriented" at the time. She also said, "I did not aim the gun. I put my hand under the pillow and fired it in a flat position." Her offer to testify in support of the present case was denied.

The prosecution's case rested on two arguments. The first was motivation based on a history of the defendant being abusive to his wife and children, and her intention to leave him. This was supported by an undated note found by the police in the wife's handbag stating her plan to take the children and leave him after the holidays. (The shooting took place on December 26.) A sleep expert was asked by the prosecution to review the prior sleep studies for evidence of a confusional arousal, and to render an opinion as to the possibility of this being an accidental shooting in a sleepwalking arousal. His opinion was that he found no evidence in the sleep studies supporting a NREM parasomnia, and that although he had no doubt the accused suffered severe OSA, there were no other cases in the scholarly literature of this disorder leading to violence.

That argument won the day. The prosecution's sleep expert published this case in 1995, prior to the publication of the new diagnostic research, starting in 2000, that provided better ways to elicit sleepwalking and identify the sleep pathology of low delta activity, as described earlier. In my view, this defendant deserves a rescoring of his sleep studies, which might well corroborate whether he has the underlying pathology for a NREM parasomnia.

But what about his motivation? Did he know his wife intended to leave him? There is no proof that he was aware of this, as the note was found in the wife's purse undated and probably not yet delivered. The argument by the prosecution's sleep expert, who examined the man's sleep tests but not the man himself, that this was the only case of OSA being a possible precipitant for a NREM parasomnia, was not actually valid. He missed one such case already published.

Other cases have indeed been published since then of adults with a double diagnosis of both OSA and a NREM parasomnia, and there are many cases of sleepwalking children who snore and have trouble breathing in sleep. Many of these children cease their sleepwalking following tonsillectomies, so their obstructed breathing is clearly what triggered the arousals and sleepwalks. Two of the adult cases were observed to arouse abruptly into parasomnia behavior while in the laboratory during a trial of CPAP to control their sleep apnea. It is clear now that even subtle difficulties in breathing during sleep can trigger a NREM parasomnia event in a vulnerable person. But could their behavior be as dangerous as to risk the shooting of a spouse?

Another case of OSA and NREM parasomnia, published in 2005, was one seen in our own laboratory, and is most closely analogous to the man who shot his wife. Our patient's NREM parasomnia problem did not emerge secondarily to the OSA during a CPAP treatment; rather, it was the primary reason for her seeking help. The patient's medical history included well-controlled hypertension and a seizure disorder that was also well-controlled. Her NREM parasomnia behaviors had begun 5 years before we saw her. She first fell asleep in her car while waiting for her daughter, awakening to find herself driving 3 miles away in a busy intersection. This occurred, she reported, about five times a month for the next 5 years. Sometimes she awoke to horns honking at her, miles from home. She also found herself barefoot in the snow in a neighbor's backyard, and once the police found her wandering in a neighboring town. She had been putting on weight and snoring, and her daytime sleepiness had also been escalating.

The incident that brought her to the Sleep Center was her worst. The woman fell asleep about 10 P.M., after watching a horror movie. She woke at 6 A.M. with her hands covered in dried blood. Next, she found blood in the kitchen on her cutting board, and then the remains of her cat next to the trash can. That did it.

This patient's sleep test showed severe OSA, which was eliminated with CPAP treatment. She has been free of sleep-related driving, wandering, and violence episodes since then. Like the man who shot his wife, she killed first, then was diagnosed with OSA. She was not charged, of course, as her victim was only a cat. Neither person had any memory of their attack, nor did either attempt to cover it up. It was probably easier for the jury to convict the man because of his apparent "motive"—that his wife was about to leave him—than to believe the complicated testimony about two sleep disorders. No one examined the man's state of mind. Would he have been better off with a psychiatric evaluation in addition to the work of the pulmonologist who testified for the defense? We may never know.

Prior to the era of sleep medicine as a distinct field of specialized knowledge, lawyers most often did turn to psychiatrists for help in clarifying the guilt or innocence of those who committed crimes while in an apparently strange state of mind. Consider the man who was found standing naked on a main thoroughfare, drinking a beer in the early morning hours. Once it was established that he was not drunk, the question was whether he suffered from a mental disorder. Was this a psychotic episode, a dissociative disorder, or fugue state? Of course, some who behave in peculiar ways do have psychiatric or neurological diagnoses, but those who fit the criteria of a sleep disorder diagnosis should not be forced into other diagnostic categories that do not fit. Until recently, many of these people were found guilty by reason of insanity and confined to mental institutions for indefinite terms only because of the lack of knowledge of the new sleep disorder diagnoses.

Unlike psychotic episodes and dissociative disorders, true NREM parasomnia behavior is restricted to a specific time of night (or of the sleep cycle, to be precise). They are also limited to short periods of time, and cease as soon as full consciousness returns. Again this is not so of psychiatric disorders. Nor do NREM parasomnias show the specific electroencephalographic (EEG) signs of a seizure disorder, or the cognitive dysfunction of those with neurodegenerative diseases. No wonder that, faced with the challenge of ruling out so many different diagnostic possibilities, many sleep experts flatly decline to serve in court cases.

A major problem until very recently was that the standard sleep laboratory testing was of little use in providing evidence of a NREM parasomnia unless an arousal from delta sleep happened to occur *during the night of the study*. It is not surprising that the expert who reviewed the sleep studies of the man who shot his wife found no such evidence. There is no validated marker in the standardized scoring of a clinical polysomnography (PSG) study—nothing like the early REM of major depression, the bursts of activity in the calf muscles detected by electromyographic (EMG) monitors that identify periodic limb movement disorder (PLMD), the pauses in breathing of ten or more seconds that mark OSA—that proves beyond a doubt that a NREM parasomnia is present. Without such evidence, sleep clinicians who attempted to defend an accused sleepwalker had to rely on their own clinical judgment, based on the patient's history of such events, a similar history in other family members, a clean police record, and the patient's believability and reputation. The Bonkalo criteria, as described previously, were also useful. Few of those accused with sleepwalking crimes have been acquitted in a court in the United States using a sleepwalking defense when a sleep expert has testified for the prosecution. Furthermore, many accused of sleep-related crimes are represented by public defenders with little knowledge and limited resources to mount a sleepwalking defense based on research evidence.

If, during the night spent in the laboratory, no sleepwalking occurs, can we not simply keep testing until we catch an episode on video tape? Unfortunately, this is not financially feasible. Sleep testing is expensive because it is labor intensive. It takes about 10 hours of a well-trained sleep technician's time to prepare a sleep subject for the night, affixing the monitors, testing that they are recording well with the patient's cooperation before saying good night. The technician must then watch the recording and the video monitor for the next 7 hours; 420 minutes of sleep is the standard duration of a clinical sleep test. Then there is the time involved in compiling data from the night into a diagnostic report. The equipment for sleep recording includes software for scoring the stages of sleep and counting the number of abnormal events in each half minute of the night. Before scoring, these recordings are always edited to remove any so-called "artifacts" (if the sleeper turns over in bed, for example, muscle activity temporarily obscures the brainwave recording during that time). Once that editing is done and the study is scored, it is independently reviewed by the sleep clinician or physician who ordered the test. That person also checks the scoring before signing off on the report.

What about home monitoring with a video camera? Would that be a cheaper solution? This technique has been tried and judged not reliable enough. The sleeper may get up to walk to the bathroom, fully awake. It is difficult to distinguish a true parasomnia from a normal awakening unless we can see that it is an arousal from delta sleep, and that the sleeper is in a confused state. Home monitoring with brainwave recording is an option, but a trained technician should be present to make repairs or perform maintenance as needed—if, for example, an electrode comes loose. This makes home studies almost as expensive as those conducted in the laboratory.

Is all of this attention warranted when violent sleepwalkers are so few? Is there any reason to think these incidents are on the rise? We do not know; in fact, sleep researchers are as a group concerned about the many who may need help but who have not applied for it. There are indirect indications that the number of sleepwalking incidents following the ingestion of one of the newer sleep medications may be increasing rapidly. Undeniably, there has been a marked explosion of blogs reporting strange behaviors in relation to taking Ambien to induce sleep. A *New York Times* story, published on March 8 2006, reported that 26.5 million prescriptions of Ambien were written in 2005, and that this drug tops the list of those found in impaired drivers' bloodstreams. The state of Washington reported 78 impaired driving arrests due to Ambien in 2005, up from 56 in 2004. Sales revenue of Ambien reached $2.2 billion in 2005. So, what we can say with certainty is that the number of sleep-related prescription, accidents, and incidents—all fitting the description of unawareness at the time of the episode and no memory of it afterward—is definitely growing. Police and other observers describe those sleepwalking on Ambien as glassy-eyed, with blank expressions; this despite having engaged in very dangerous behavior.

There has been no large epidemiologic study of the presence of parasomnias in the general public since 1997, when a survey study was conducted in the United Kingdom of close to 5,000 people between the ages of 15 and 100. The 2,078 men and 2,894 women were questioned by telephone by a trained interviewer using a standardized questionnaire. The survey focused only on sleep-related violence. A total of 106 respondents reported that they were currently experiencing violent behaviors during sleep—2.1% of the sample. If we multiply this by the population in the United States, we have a lot of potential trouble. If we include with those the newer diagnoses of sleep eating, exploring and sleep sex, the percentage of people afflicted with NREM parasomnias might reach as high as 10% of adults.

Who were those in the survey who reported violent episodes? More were males (2.6%) than females (1.7%). Three percent were between 15 and 44 years old. The rate dropped to 0.4% in those 65 or older. Most were married, 54%, so they had a confirming partner who was also a potential target. Most partners had taken to sleeping in another room or had sent the violent sleeper to spend the night elsewhere, behind a locked door.

Comparing those who reported they were violent in sleep to those who were not turned up some important differences. The violent ones complained of more insomnia of all types—getting to sleep, staying asleep, and waking too early without being able to return to sleep—suggesting they were chronically sleep deprived. We know this is a risk factor for abnormal arousals. Why were they having so much trouble getting a good night of sleep? The violent sleepers had a greater prevalence of a mood or anxiety disorder diagnosis than did those with no violence. They also reported more often that they snored and had symptoms of sleep apnea, as well as of excessive limb movements during sleep (70%). In other words, the violent sleepers had less sleep, and the sleep they did get was disrupted by pauses in breathing and leg movements. They also used caffeine to excess (which is disruptive of slow-wave sleep [SWS]), consuming six or more cups of caffeinated beverages a day, perhaps to ward off the sleepiness following their poor nights of sleep. Many more reported vivid hallucinations at sleep onset, most often feeling that they were about to be attacked. There were no reports of these experiences from the nonviolent respondents. These data help to fill in the picture of the interaction of waking emotional difficulties (mood and anxiety disorders) with the normal processes of sleep, disrupting sleep especially in those who have excessive movements or who may be short of breath. Sleepless nights will be followed by sleepiness next day and often the over-use of caffeine, which is, in turn, disruptive to the next night's sleep. A vicious cycle is set in motion, leading to abrupt arousals into unconscious defensive or protective behaviors—without any critical judgment operating to test the reality of the perceived threat.

This information reveals potentially defining characteristics of those who face prosecution for an act they cannot remember but that may have been motivated by a basic sense of threat, even by the very state of sleep itself. All things considered, it takes a lot of trust to lay limply unconscious for several hours, perhaps beside another person, off guard to the dangers of predation. We humans have probably inherited some sense of risk in connection with sleeping from our prehistoric ancestors, who slept unprotected on the open savannahs. I noted earlier that this sleep anxiety appears to be heightened when we sleep more lightly due to some ongoing stress, or attempt to sleep in an unfamiliar bed. Consider the young man who had a violent episode while sleeping in the guest room of his fiancée's parents' home. It was their first meeting, and he was trying to make a good impression by being on his best behavior. He got up from sleep and knocked all the pictures off the walls causing a great crash and much broken glass. Parents who are aware of the sense of threat in a child's awakenings sometimes try to address the fear with the night-time prayer, "Now I lay me down to sleep . . . ," although this may not work to reassure the child that they will be safe in God's hands, given the last line, "If I should die before I wake . . ."

Where We Are Now

The two new diagnostic advances described earlier, the spectral analysis scoring (showing that true sleepwalkers have significantly lower than normal delta activity in the first sleep cycle) and the new sleep-deprivation protocol with increasingly louder auditory tones, are both very useful in identifying the true sleepwalker. The new, finer grained scoring of SWS identifies the underlying neurological disorder as one of easy arousability from delta sleep. The sleep-deprivation protocol acts as a clinical probe, provoking an actual behavioral arousal under laboratory conditions. Although a series of studies were published on these methods between 2000 and 2008, they have not yet been adopted as being the officially sanctioned diagnostic tools. Acceptance of new diagnostic methods in sleep medicine—as in all areas of medicine—is a slow process, and one accompanied by a good deal of skepticism and reluctance. This is frustrating to lawyers and families trying to help someone in trouble.

The "state of mind" at the time of a sleepwalking event, particularly a violent one, is a tricky issue. We can produce sleepwalking behavior in true sleepwalkers and diagnose them with NREM parasomnia, but this still leaves the question of what was on the sleepwalkers' minds before falling asleep on the night of a violent arousal. This is the old question of motivation, whether conscious or unconscious. Even if we can prove that the person has the hallmark low delta activity in sleep that is a condition for easy arousability, why don't they just go back to sleep instead of getting into trouble? Must there be a "prepared mind" leading the sleeper to misperceive and react as if to a threat?

How can we be sure that the person charged with a sleepwalking crime did not plan the attack, was not fully conscious while it was committed? This problem is particularly sticky when a sleep expert for the prosecution argues that the defendant was fully awake, as was the case in the Falater murder trial. One leader in the sleep medicine field has written strongly and often, urging there be no involvement of sleep experts in court cases on either side. His point is that we cannot know the state of mind at the time violence occurs, and so should stay away from lending any opinion on the matter.

Now that our diagnostic tools are able to produce clearer evidence of whether a person is vulnerable to acting aggressively or sexually due to a specific sleep disorder, will some who were convicted of sleep-related crimes prior to the development of these new techniques be allowed to petition to have a new study, or a new trial? After all, DNA testing, when it became available, led to the exoneration of many people wrongly convicted of crimes. The NREM parasomnia cases are a bit different—the defendant did the deed, but without the necessary mental awareness or intent to establish culpability.

The Hammer Man, as I call him, is one such case. He is serving a life sentence for a nonlethal physical attack on the teenaged son of his girlfriend. The man had been sleeping in the living room when he was aroused by the boy. He picked up a hammer he had been using before sleep, which was lying beside him. He grabbed it by the head and hit the boy a "glancing" blow with the handle. He was convicted of assault with intent to murder, and received the life sentence without parole.

The Hammer Man had been imprisoned for 5 years when he petitioned for a sleep study on the grounds that he had been denied the testing before his conviction. The appeal was granted, and he was released for 2 days so that he could be tested under the newly published sleep-deprivation guidelines. With his lawyer, I arranged for a local sleep expert to carry out the testing and to have the Hammer Man's delta (SWS) activity scoring be done by an independent expert—the first sleep researcher in the United States to publish the results of this more refined scoring method that distinguishes sleepwalkers from non-walkers. Christian Guilleminault, a senior sleep researcher at Stanford University, followed his initial 2001 study with a series of research studies using spectral analysis scoring of both children and adults. He is the leading expert in this country on this scoring method as applied to NREM parasomnias.

The first sleep study night showed the Hammer Man to have moderately severe OSA. This was an unanticipated finding. In addition, the report of his brain wave recording states that the Hammer Man had extremely low delta activity in the first sleep cycle. This means he was vulnerable to an abnormal arousal from the first hour of sleep into a mixed state of partial waking and partial sleep. Given that he was also positive for obstructed breathing, it is likely that his aggressive act was caused by his confused mental state after he was disturbed by the boy. He did not show any attempt to sleepwalk while being sleep tested, but as a convicted prisoner he was chained to the bed with shackles that restricted his ability to move.

What was on his mind the night he attacked the boy? His felt his whole world had just collapsed. He was divorced, and his former wife had kept the family house in the settlement. The Hammer Man had just heard that she was about to sell the house and relocate out of state, taking their children with her. He would no longer be able to visit them regularly, and this was a major loss to him. Further adding to his despair, his girlfriend broke off their engagement and told him that she was preparing to leave the country permanently, taking her two teenage boys with her. She also told him to leave the house, but he had no place to go. He was devastated, and begged to stay the night. On top of this was an ongoing third problem, financial difficulties with his business, that was causing him to lose sleep. After an emotionally stormy night of tears and fears of abandonment, he dropped into an immediate deep sleep on the living room couch. He awoke still holding the hammer he had been using that evening to help his girlfriend pack up boxes for her move. He had no memory of having struck the boy with the handle.

The results of the Hammer Man's sleep study were presented by his new defense lawyer at a hearing before the judge who had sentenced him, along with a request for the judge to consider an acquittal or a retrial. At the time of this writing, no judgment had yet been rendered. If this case has a positive outcome (for the Hammer Man), it may set a precedent that will surely be followed with other such requests. If the evidence of the Hammer Man's underlying delta sleep pathology and possible abnormal sleep apnea–related arousal, along with his desperately unhappy state of mind, are seen as factors mitigating his guilt, this may form the basis for a release for time served. It is even possible that this case, together with the recent acquittal also based partly on the low delta activity of the Good Neighbor, the man who entered his neighbor's home, could prompt the reopening of other cases, including perhaps Scott Falater's.

Sleep Experts Disagree

The disagreement between the prosecution and defense sleep experts in the Falater case is not over; a continuing dialogue between us now involves a widening group of others. One venue is in professional journals that reflect two different models of the disorder underlying the abnormal arousal in sleepwalking; another is the legal arena. These two battlegrounds are intimately connected.

A basic problem is that American courts are set up to be adversarial in nature, each side may be motivated more to win than to seek the truth. We have made progress in identifying the presence of a neurological difference in the SWS of those exhibiting NREM parasomnia behavior, but we have not solved the problem of how to establish certainty about the sleepwalker's state of mind, or even the state of the state—asleep versus awake—during the time the specific behavior took place. This has caused a former president of the American Academy of Sleep Medicine to warn over and over that sleep experts should not become advocates but should rather offer the same opinion to either side as a service to the court. This is an ideal that will be difficult to apply in U.S. courts.

Of course, sleep experts have the option when asked to accept or refuse to testify, but the decision should be based on their professional judgment of the validity of the case. I believe that when we take an oath as responsible, well-trained, board-certified sleep clinicians, we can and should lend our expertise to interpret facts in an unbiased manner for the benefit of a jury. Furthermore, I believe it is a good bargain; even though unpaid I have gained a lot of information in return for services rendered. I feel strongly that we should not deny our help to a person in trouble, provided we do not stray beyond our knowledge base and into the realm of speculation.

Helpful guidelines are available for keeping these boundaries in mind. One is the recently published CHESS method. This is a framework to which the evidence for and against the defendant meeting the criteria of a NREM parasomnia can be applied, organized, and weighed, using knowledge of the current research literature; previously published cases; one's own experience with diagnostic possibilities of neurological, psychiatric, and substance effects producing similar symptoms; and, of course, the defendant's own and family history of sleep disorders. The formula helps experts remain unbiased and is comprised of five steps:

C: Formulating an initial opinion or Claim
H: Establishing a Hierarchy of supporting evidence
E: Examining the Evidence
S: Studying the evidence
S: Synthesizing a revised opinion

Next, a judgment must be reached as to whether it is highly unlikely, likely, or highly likely that the defendant was in a state of nonconsciousness during the specific crime with which they are charged (or that there is insufficient data to assess the likelihood). This is the basis for rendering an independent opinion, and I have used it to assess those cases on which I have been asked to consult.

As a clinician, I enjoy helping patients. I do not enjoy testifying in court. Standing up to a smart prosecutor or defense lawyer while they try to shake my testimony can be challenging. I do enjoy the outcome of an acquittal when I am convinced that the defendant's action was due to an underlying sleep disorder and a nonconscious state of mind at the time. I feel great satisfaction when science and understanding trumps ignorance and skepticism.

Warnings from the Land of Nod: Nightmares and REM Behavior Disorder

Like one, that on a lonesome road
Doth walk in fear and dread
And having once turn'd round, walks on
And turns no more his head:
Because he knows, a frightful fiend
Doth close behind him tread.

—S.T. Coleridge, *The Rime of the Ancient Mariner*

When waking hours are frightening, for whatever reason, the sleeping brain may reprocess horrible images with enough raw fear attached to awaken a sleeper with a horrendous nightmare. Persistent nightmares can follow a traumatic event even in very young children. Some of the preschoolers who witnessed the 9/11 Twin Tower destruction continued to have nightmares, as well as waking symptoms of anxiety and depression, for years after the towers came down. The researchers who followed them up found an interesting difference between those children who had these long-lasting effects and those who did not: Those who experienced anxiety and nightmares had also experienced some previous frightening event like a dog bite, a car accident, or tonsillectomy. Children with no previous history of trauma were free of these effects.

Earlier scary incidents can leave behind memories of a frightening sudden threat to the integrity of the self. If these are followed by another fear-inducing event, and if there have not been other, more positive memories for the youngster to draw on and from which to create dreams that down-regulate the threat during the night, children may be left with reactivated scary memories that provide the images for frightening dream scenarios. How much worse off are those whose daily conditions of living involve unpredictable, ongoing traumatic events as inescapable as war? An abusive parent or spouse, and prolonged imprisonment with or without torture, are other examples of such conditions. The common feature is a threat of harm, accompanied by a lack of ability to control the circumstances of the threat, and the lack of or inability to develop protective behaviors.

Which strategies are best for coping effectively under circumstances of extreme stress and fear has been controversial among those who have researched and written about this issue. Is denial of the threatening event, and avoidance of thoughts about it, a better strategy than being vigilant and sensitized to what is going on, and its implications for one's survival?

Denial was once thought to be the healthiest coping strategy for those who had survived the Holocaust and immigrated to Israel. Some 40 years after the end of World War II, a group of survivors was recruited for a study that compared the sleep and dreams of those who were well-adjusted in their waking lives to those who were not; a third group of controls were native-born Israelis free of traumatic experiences. The volunteers spent 5 nights being recorded in a sleep laboratory. The well-adjusted Holocaust survivors had dramatically fewer dreams that they could recall than did the other two groups; only 33% of their awakenings from rapid eye movement (REM) sleep yielded a dream report. Those who were poorly adjusted recalled dreams 55% of the time they were awakened, and the nontraumatized native-born group had 78% recall. What they dreamed about was even more surprising. The well-adjusted survivors had short everyday dreams of trivial subjects that were without emotion. The poorly adjusted survivors had more anxiety dreams, some that were true nightmares, recapitulating their experiences under the threat of the Gestapo. The sleep of both the well-adjusted émigrés and the native-born controls was of equally good quality but the poorly adjusted survivors had trouble getting to sleep and had many awakenings during the night.

The conclusion drawn by the authors of that study was that the well-adjusted survivors used a denial technique both day and night that was protective against the intrusion of horrific experiences as memories, which would not help their waking adjustment to their new circumstances. Their poor recall rate was associated with their very deep sleep, and the high rate of recall of those with poor adaptation was attributed to their very light sleep. The study was controversial at the time it was published in 1991, as it appeared to praise "erasing" frightening memories as a healthy response to emotional trauma. My own comment at the time was that the study took place so long after the traumatic event (the Holocaust itself) that it could not really speak to whether the well-adjusted had perhaps had very different dreams closer to the time of the trauma. Perhaps they had had emotional dreams that down-regulated their anxiety and fear across the night, with plots that linked the current negative images to previous more positive images to change their coping strategies productively. If the well-adjusted survivors had not just buried access to the memories but instead had put them into their long-term memory networks in association with more positive recent experiences, that would support this as a healthy mechanism. However, I was skeptical that all was well with the so called "well-adjusted" survivors, due to their abnormally low recall rate of dreams from REM awakenings. When all is well in waking life, research has shown, dream recall is usually at 80%—just as it was for the native-born controls.

One clear principle that comes out of this work is that the effects of trauma on sleep and dreaming depend on the nature of the threat. If direct action against the threat is irrelevant or impossible (as it would be if the trauma was well in the past), then denial may be helpful in reducing stress so that the person can get on with living as best they can. However, if the threat will be encountered over and over (such as with spousal abuse), and direct action would be helpful in addressing the threat, then denial by avoiding thinking about the danger (which helps in the short-term) will undermine problem-solving efforts and mastery in the long run. In other words, if nothing can be done, emotion-coping efforts to regulate the distress (dreaming) is a good strategy; but if constructive actions can be taken, waking problem-solving action is more adaptive.

Where do nightmares fit into this thinking? Nightmares are defined as frightening dreams that wake the sleeper into full consciousness and with a clear memory of the dream imagery. These are not to be confused with sleep terrors. There are three main differences between these two. First, nightmare arousals are more often from late in the night's sleep, when dreams are longest and the content is most bizarre and affect-laden (emotional); sleep terrors occur early in sleep. Second, nightmares are REM sleep-related, while sleep terrors come out of non-REM (NREM) slow-wave sleep (SWS). Third, sleepers experience vivid recall of nightmares, whereas with sleep terrors the experience is of full or partial amnesia for the episode itself, and only rarely is a single image recalled.

If we are right that the mind is continuously active throughout sleep— reviewing emotion-evoking new experiences from the day, scanning memory networks for similar experiences (which will defuse immediate emotional impact), revising by updating our organized sense of ourselves, and rehearsing new coping behaviors—nightmares are an exception and fail to perform these functions. Nightmares that wake the sleeper abort the completion of the REM dream. Waking up may relieve the sleeper's negative emotion, temporarily. ("I am not about to be eaten by a monster. I am safe in my own bed.") But if the fear-invoking waking situation is ongoing, the nightmare itself will be of no help in regulating emotions unless and until new waking experiences occur that have successful outcomes and that are then filed into long-term memory. This explains why nightmares are more common in youngsters (estimates of their frequency run all the way from 5% to 30%), and gradually decline in frequency as children learn how to manage waking negative experiences by developing real coping skills for resolving their fears.

Not everyone has nightmares, and those who do experience a wide range of frequency of these sleep-disturbing dreams. The negative emotion that precipitates the awakening is not always fear; in some cases it is anger, disgust, or grief that induces the arousal. Surveys asking about the once-a-week frequency of this problem find that nightmares peak in the mid teenage years and then drop to between 2% and 6% of the adult general public. These numbers are based on retrospective reports, meaning that those being surveyed were asked, "Do you have nightmares, and if so how frequently?" When people are asked instead to keep logs of their nightly dreams and to note which are nightmares, a prospective approach, then the rates of reported nightmares are higher. Both of these methods of investigation indicate that women suffer from nightmares at a much higher rate than men, a ratio of about 4:1. This should not be a surprise, given that women are higher reporters of dreams generally, and also that they have higher rates of insomnia and disorders that have to do with emotion regulation. It follows then that women are more often diagnosed with major depression and with anxiety disorders than are men.

Adults who report nightmares almost always (80%–98% of the time) claim to have suffered from them in childhood as well. Half of a group of teenagers who were studied over a 3-year period, from when they were 15 to the age of 18, reported no change in nightmare frequency. But this figure masked a big gender difference. Girls had an increasing frequency of nightmares over this time period, while the frequency in boys was decreasing. In sum, nightmares appear to be more common in those who have intense reactions to stress. The criteria cited for nightmare disorder in the diagnostic manual for psychiatric disorders, the *Diagnostic and Statistical Manual IV-TR* (DSM IV-TR), include this phrase "frightening dreams usually involving threats to survival, security, or self-esteem." This theme may sound familiar: Remember that threats to self-esteem seem to precede NREM parasomnia awakenings. All of this is evidence that the mind, although asleep, is constantly concerned about the safety and integrity of the self.

Help for the Nightmare Sufferer

It seems that there are various weak points in the mechanism responsible for switching between sleeping and waking throughout the regular changes of states of the 24-hour cycle. Under conditions of persistent stress, the introduction or excessive use of some medication or substance, or the development of a breathing disorder of sleep, these weak points break down and a sleep disorder becomes manifest. When sleep is interrupted by an arousal, the successful completion of the work of the night mind is interrupted, and the reduction of negative emotion is halted. One of these underlying weak points, responsible for arousals from both NREM and REM sleep, is of genetic origin. This has been proven with studies of twins, both identical (monozygotic) and fraternal (dizygotic) pairs. One large twin study found that people are six times more likely to have a NREM parasomnia (either sleepwalking or sleep terrors) if their identical twins also have the disorder than are those whose nonidentical twins have the disorder. Twin study evidence and family history studies also show a strong contribution of genetics to adult nightmares.

Besides genetics, other factors hypothesized to contribute to adult nightmares are poor sleep hygiene (irregular sleep hours) and an avoidant style of thinking about nightmare images. Although we cannot change a person's genes (yet), we can reduce the impact of the other two: educational programs have been designed to control or reduce the frequency of nightmares by focusing on sleep hygiene—stressing the importance of keeping to a regular sleep schedule and getting enough hours of sleep. Other therapeutic techniques focus on active confrontation of the nightmare images by rehearsing them while awake. Some studies have compared these techniques—nightmare imagery rehearsal during waking and training in a physical relaxation technique. It appears from a review of the few such formal studies that rehearsal of nightmare images is more effective than is just recording them in a log combined with learning to relax. Rehearsal during the day with active instruction on how to change the ending of the nightmare is more effective than is passive rehearsal. More well-controlled studies are needed to address this, so that clinicians can offer the best treatments.

I have used a somewhat different approach with patients whose nightmares are severe in frequency and impacting their waking lives. As one may guess,

I focus on the night. One beautiful young woman asked for help with night-mares that occurred not just nightly but several times each night. The night-mares were accompanied by intense fear, high heart rate, and a drenching perspiration. She would have to change her nightgown to be able to get back to sleep. Sometimes the physiological effect was so strong that she had to change her bed sheets as well. This had been going on for years, but she was finally brought to seek help after getting married; she wanted to be able to sleep peace-fully (and dry) with her husband.

As a rather flamboyant fun-loving teenager, this woman had attracted men's interest and, on two occasions, was overpowered and raped. These were the traumas behind the nightmares. She had become sexually closed off and for that reason had put off marriage until her mid-thirties. Her husband was unde-manding and patient with her.

We started her treatment with a night in the Sleep Disorder Service labora-tory to collect dreams from her REM periods; we would be working directly with these in her treatment program. As so often happens, the patient had a better night in the lab than she usually experienced at home. We were able to record three dreams that were not of nightmare severity. These gave us a chance to look into how she saw herself in her dreams, and together we began to work out the dimensions of her self-concept, the polarities by which she defined her-self in relation to others. These were: smart–dumb, hardworking–lazy, active-passive, ethical–sneaky, warm–cold, and attractive–ugly, in her first dreams. She saw herself as mostly on the positive side of these dimensions. She was smart, hardworking, ethical, and attractive, but also passive and cold. I asked her to have her husband sleep separately for the first few weeks of her treat-ment, so that she would be relieved of the anxiety of disturbing his sleep. Her homework from Session One was to remember that she was the author of her dreams, and since she had made them up, she was to remind herself that she could also learn to take control of them and make them end more positively. She was to keep a log of remembered dreams and to note whether or not they woke her in fear. She caught on quickly and, in Session Two, she related an interesting first successful ending to a scary dream.

"I was lying on my back on the floor of an open elevator that was rising above the city of Chicago. I was alone and scared that this was dangerous. It kept going higher and higher. I decided to get up to see where I was, and as I did that the elevator walls slid up to protect me." She was very excited about this dream, seeing that when, instead of being passive, she had taken action and, as she put it, "when I stood up for myself," she was safe and felt okay.

This was a short treatment program. In only five sessions, the patient had mastered four important steps in using her dream log to improve her sleep: (1) *R*eviewing her dream log to identify the negative feeling, behavior, or trait that she was experiencing; (2) *I*dentifying when an ongoing dream was becoming scary; (3) *S*topping the dream even if she had to force her eyes open; and (4) *C*hanging the negative aspect to a positive one in her dreams. I call this the RISC method, an acronym to remind patients to take a chance on being active on their own behalf. This particular patient learned quickly to stop those dreams that were becoming frightening. In one dream, she was at a cocktail party and a man there began to hassle her, moving in too close, backing her into an isolated corner. She told me with a grin, "I stopped that scenario and next saw myself sitting across the breakfast table telling my sister about that party." She was using avoidance as her coping technique rather than problem-solving, but she did abort the fear and stayed safely asleep.

When I called the patient a year after she had terminated treatment, I was told she was no longer at the office where she had worked. I was concerned that perhaps things had gotten worse for her. I called her home phone number. She answered and was happy to tell me she had taken a break from working in order to care for her newborn. That was great news for her to share. "But how are the nightmares?" I asked. She said she rarely had one, and when she did she was able to decode and correct it quickly. Although her symptoms were initially severe, she was an easy case in treatment. This is not always the case.

Post-traumatic Stress Disorder Nightmares

Nightmares, a symptom of post-traumatic stress disorder (PTSD), are categorized separately from idiopathic nightmares (the term *idiopathic* indicates that we have no clue where they came from). The patient just discussed had experienced a real trauma that initiated the nightmares, but she did not have the waking symptoms of PTSD. Perhaps she could have had a mild case of PTSD, although her nighttime disruptions were far from mild. In any case, in PTSD we can point to a horrendous event as the source of the nightmares, either of a personal or a shared experience, and to waking symptoms that are part of the diagnostic criteria for this disorder (and which are not present in the idiopathic nightmare sufferer). These include symptoms commonly called *flashbacks*, intrusions of images of the traumatic event during the day either as a vivid recollection of the event, or the sense that the event is actually occurring again. These reliving episodes may last only a few seconds or as long as days, according to the DSM-IV-TR. Another symptom is what is known as "numbing," a reduction of responsiveness. This includes avoidance of anything that reminds the sufferer of the traumatic event, including talking about it with others, and even some reduced recall of important aspects of what happened. There is also increased arousal—a sort of hypervigilance, or an expectation of trouble, with an exaggerated startle response to a sudden loud noise or touch.

The sleep and dreaming symptoms of PTSD are also described as more severe than those of the idiopathic nightmare type. In fact, they are considered by some experts to be a third type of dreaming disorder, distinct from both REM nightmares and from NREM night terrors, which most often arise from delta sleep. These PTSD nightmares arise typically from both REM and Stage 2 sleep, the light sleep stage that occupies 50% of the night, but they can occur within any sleep stage. This suggests that when negative emotional experience is strong enough, a serious threat to the integrity of body and soul, all of sleep may be vulnerable to repeated image reminders of earlier traumatic events. In men, the trauma is most often that of military combat, while in women it is intimate partner violence and violent injury, often during a sexual assault.

The primary sleep symptom of PTSD is insomnia, but sleep apnea, periodic limb movements of sleep (PLMS), sleep talking, and hypnagogic and hypno-pompic hallucinations (sensory images at the onset of sleep and coincident with the morning awakening) have all been reported as troublesome symptoms. This shows that a good deal of both sleep disturbance and active image-production is going on throughout the night. No wonder a high rate of major depression and alcohol abuse is associated with PTSD; alcohol and substance use have been interpreted as an attempt to self-medicate, to blot out awareness of the distressing images and feelings. The presence of specific sleep disorders—insomnia, PLMS, and sleep apnea—in PTSD patients has been considered secondary and has not received the focused attention it deserves. A recent scholarly review of this issue makes a strong case that, unless treated, disturbed sleep will persist, even after successful treatment of the nightmares. It is likely that insomnia is a precondition for PTSD, and its treatment should be incorporated into any program addressing the nightmares. Those who treat these patients must follow up with them, even with those who have gained so-called successful control of their nightmares, to ensure that these other sleep disorders are under control. Otherwise, they may continue to undermine the peace of the night.

Now, what about the mind? What can we deduce about it from the night-mares themselves? Again, we find emotion at the core of nightmares—in this case fear amounting to terror. Distinctive about nightmares is the repetitious nature of their content; these dreams are almost like a broken record, stuck in a groove and unable to play on, or rather play out, by relating the trauma experi-ence to other memory material that might help defuse the impact of the over-whelming emotion. This pattern of dreaming is called the *repetitive-traumatic pattern* and is in contrast to the *progressive-sequential pattern*, in which dreams evolve and change over time.

Not all PTSD sufferers have the repetitive nightmare type. One well-done study compared three groups of Vietnam veterans. In Group 1, nightmares had started only after a combat experience, and each person in this group had a clear PTSD diagnosis. Group 2 was made up of veterans with a lifelong history of nightmares but with no combat experience. Group 3 had heavy combat experience but no nightmares—these were the control subjects. All were studied about 8 years after their return from the war. The nightmares of the first group differed from those of the second dramatically. All of those whose nightmares started after their combat experience had the repetitive pattern, with almost the exact same dream over and over; furthermore, what they dreamed was a replication of an actual event. The nightmares of this first group started early in the night's sleep and continued throughout the night. None of the veterans in Group 2, who had lifelong histories of nightmares, experienced the replication of an actual event, and their nightmares did not show the repetitive dream pattern. Instead they had long, frightening dreams with varied stories. When the dreams did include combat scenarios, they were not of events that had actually been experienced. These nightmares occurred late in the night. The first group responded well to psychotherapy; the second did not.

There were similarities in the backgrounds of the men in Groups 1 and 3, those with clear PTSD and the controls. Most members of both groups had fairly normal childhood and adolescent histories—quite different from those in Group 2, the lifelong nightmare group. Most of the men in Group 2 shared an interesting distinctive feature: They lacked girlfriends or other close friends, and had poor academic histories. They tended to be isolated, some had artistic interests.

Other research supports the profile of the PTSD sufferer described by this study; having had more severe combat exposure, the men of Group 1, who had PTSD, had fewer emotional resources with which to cope. They were younger than those not affected by PTSD, less educated, and had often experienced the loss of a close friend in combat. These characteristics are in contrast to the combat controls, who described their survival tactic as learning quickly not to get too close, or dependent, on anyone while in Vietnam.

Another interesting finding reported in several studies is that chronic nightmare sufferers do not typically begin having nightmares immediately after a combat event but some time later, following another trauma involving the loss of a relationship or rejection. (This is also true of the 9/11 children who continued to suffer nightmares. They too had experienced an earlier trauma.) The veteran who suffers the breakup of a marriage on returning home, for example, may then begin to experience nightmares. The nightmare is often not about the current loss experience, but this trauma revives the older wartime imagery, demonstrating that present traumatic experiences are linked in dreaming to similar older memories. Remember that the studies of dreams and depression related to divorce found that when the dream narrative linked the present upsetting event to past emotionally related memories, this indicated that a therapeutic process was under way that would reduce the impact of the trauma over time.

Nightmares and REM Behavior Disorder

Another group of patients who experience a behavioral arousal out of REM sleep are distinct from those with idiopathic nightmares and from PTSD patients, both of whom awaken and orient quickly to reality in a fully conscious state. This new group of sleepers arise from REM and actually act out their dreams. They were first studied by the sleep team of Mark Mahowald and Carlos Schenck of the Hennepin County sleep program in Minneapolis. They observed these patients were most often elderly persons suffering from some neurological damage that allowed movement to occur during REM sleep. Normally, such movement is prevented by inhibition of the spinal motor nerves, keeping the sleeper in a state of muscle paralysis as long as the REM period lasts. These sleepers were described as "leaping from bed, punching and kicking and causing repeated injury in violent confrontations with dream characters." They were not seizure-related episodes, nor were these psychiatric patients. In fact, most often these were very pleasant, mild-mannered men, somewhat embarrassed by their nocturnal behaviors as described to their doctors by their spouses. Bed partners reported they had suffered injuries from these bouts. Fractures and lacerations followed dreams of being attacked or chased and occasionally of hunting, being in combat, or playing football.

The sleep of those suffering from *REM behavior disorder* (RBD) is distinctive. It shows muscle twitching activity in both arms and legs, occurring in both NREM and REM sleep. The normal loss of muscle tone during REM is intermittent in these people, failing to persist throughout the REM sleep period. The chin monitors worn by these patients during sleep show bursts of muscle activity. The behavioral acting out is so vigorous in some of these cases that patients develop their own ways of controlling themselves. Some sleep zipped up in a sleeping bag, others tie themselves to a bed post and remove all breakable objects from the vicinity before sleep. The vivid dreams they act out may involve shooting a deer or tackling in football. Aggressive behaviors often have a theme we have encountered before: "Something is going to hurt my family, and I am trying to protect them."

Early on in the work-up of these patients signs of some neurodegenerative disorders, primarily of the Parkinson's type were observed but multiple system atrophy and dementia with Lewy body disease have also been implicated. Studies have shown that the RBD sleep symptoms often *precede* any apparent waking mental deterioration. This early warning sign offers an advantage in that whatever treatment is available can be started early. Recall we have also seen this before; sleep problems precede other health issues, as in those suffering chronic insomnia, where the poor sleep is an early warning sign for major depression. Sleep symptoms are often the first indication of some trouble not yet apparent during waking hours; this makes their early identification and treatment that much more important.

One of my students, a handsome, smart young man, came to see me with what he had diagnosed for himself as a "dream enactment" problem. This, he said, had started just 3 months before, with no earlier history of any sleep disorder. He was physically healthy, on no medications, did not smoke, and drank alcohol rarely. He was doing well in his academic program and was also happily married. I asked him next how often this dream enactment was occurring and was surprised to hear that it happened about 5 out of every 7 nights a week, and frequently more than once a night. That is a lot of trouble. Next, I inquired about his memory of these events, and why he called them "dream enactments." A bit sheepishly he described his most recent performance: He suddenly sat up in bed and yelled to his wife, "You grab the tail. I'll grab the head." What was happening? He thought there was an anaconda in their bed—a very frightening experience. Next, I wanted to know if he ever got out of bed when this was happening. Again, he was a little embarrassed to tell me, "Yes. Another time I thought I was carrying the Olympic torch and marched around the bedroom." This did not sound like a sleep terror episode. Could he really have RBD at his young age of 24?

He had the clinical sleep study known as a polysomnogram, or PSG. This showed frequent short busts of muscle activity in the legs; his calf muscles twitched in both NREM and REM sleep. His REM sleep, too, did not show the normal continuous loss of muscle tone. He had increased muscle activity interrupting his REM sleep, just as an RBD patient would. The diagnosis was now either a very early warning sign of a neurodegenerative process, or something else. In our follow-up interview, I probed further for any childhood history. He told me that he was known to sleep talk and to yell out in his sleep on occasion, but not to sleepwalk or to have the panicky scream, rapid heart rate, and other signs of a sleep terror. There was no family history of NREM parasomnias, and his history was sounding without doubt like a REM sleep disorder. What else had been new in his life around the time these behaviors started 3 months ago? Two things: He had gotten married, and he had begun studying hard for his second-year board exams. Did that mean a loss of sleep? You bet!

I looked up the published studies on RBD and found no hint that stress or sleep deprivation could precipitate an RBD—at least not at this young man's age. My student met the diagnostic criteria, but his age of onset at 24 was far below the published average onset age of 53. He did show the prodrome (preliminary symptoms) of sleep talking, yelling out, and limb twitching, which again the literature indicated began an average of 22 years *before* the appearance of an RBD sleep disorder. I was reluctant to put the diagnostic label on his case and to start the usual treatment regimen of small doses of clonazepam, the drug that has proven to work well for this and the NREM parasomnias. I decided to bet that he might be able to control these events by following strict rules for sleep hygiene—no "all nighters" when cramming for exams, practicing some stress management techniques, and calling in weekly to report his sleep hours and dream enactment events. His wife promised to cooperate in reinforcing the regular sleep hours, and in keeping track of his dream enactments. Medication could always be started later if needed. A follow-up a year and a half later indicated that this patient's nights had remained peaceful.

Without a doubt, this patient had a weak spot in the sleep system of motor inhibition during both NREM and REM sleep, which allowed him to be too muscle active while asleep. This may indicate that he is in for additional trouble down the road, but if so it is a long way off. I felt this young man needed to gain the confidence that he could take care of himself and enjoy his career and personal life without feeling that a serious neurological disorder was inevitable. I may be wrong, but I trusted that the help we gave him—teaching him to honor the importance of adequate amounts of regular sleep and to handle his stress with relaxation techniques—would stand him in good stead while research into this problem progresses. It is generally true that when a new disorder is first identified, its description depends on the characteristics of those patients first diagnosed. As more patients come forth, however, we often see diagnostic criteria become both more inclusive and more differentiated. This enables us to distinguish between those with a good prognosis and a poor one.

Animal Models of REM Behavior Disorder

The major sleep failure involved in RBD is the lack of inhibition of muscle tone in REM sleep; this is the underlying pathology that allows REM dreams to be performed behaviorally. Early research done on cats helped lead sleep scientists to this finding. When sleep research was in its infancy, a search was under way for the location in the brain of the various elements of REM sleep. A pioneer in this search, and in finding the answers, was Michel Jouvet, a French neurologist. It was Jouvet who did the first innovative research in this area, and who then taught his surgical techniques to many of the American sleep researchers who traveled to France to learn from him at his laboratory in Lyon.

Jouvet describes himself as having been addicted to dreaming for close to 60 years—not just out of the desire to answer the "how does this work" questions (the mechanisms in the brain) but also the "why." Jouvet first approached the "how" surgically, trying to find what caused major muscles to stop working when dreaming began. Cats were a handy model as they, like humans, sleep a lot. They also show the same loss of postural tone when they have rapid movements of the eyes. Assuming that constructing a dream requires a high level of brain activity, Jouvet began his search for those areas of the brain involved in REM sleep by removing the cerebral cortex, which did not interfere with the onset of REM sleep. He went further and removed the hypothalamus and the pituitary gland. Again there was no effect. Periodically, the eyes would move rapidly, while breathing and heart rates speeded up. He concluded then that it was the bottom of the brain, in the brainstem—the pons and the medulla—that alone were the structures essential in the creation of REM sleep. The abrupt loss of muscle tone was prevented by a surgery Jouvet performed that separated the pons from the forebrain; all the other features of REM sleep remained present. The effect on the cats' behavior was extraordinary. Jouvet described them as "hallucinating." They raised their heads and appeared to watch something invisible, although they were not awake. Then they would arch their backs, their fur would stand up, and with no apparent provocation, they would attack some "dreamed" threat (although these were well-mannered cats when in wakefulness).

Jouvet's work has continued and has become more precise in mapping how the REM loss of muscle tone, called *atonia*, is controlled. His conclusion is that this is an active process of inhibition and not a passive lack of motor activity. The observation that the cats' behavior is in the nature of attack and defense is also helpful in understanding the observations made of human behavior in RBD patients, who engage in similar defensive aggression attacks.

Recent studies by American researcher Adrian Morrison have added to this model of RBD in the cat. When he made an additional, one-sided lesion in the central nucleus of the amygdala, the area associated with expression of fear, Morrison reported that a startle reflex to a sudden noise was released when the cat was in either NREM or REM sleep. Ordinarily, this response would only follow if the cat were awake. We know from the studies of NREM parasomnia patients that a sudden noise is also a trigger for a sleepwalking event, during which some people behave similarly to Morrison's startled cats.

What are the RBD patients dreaming? The dreams that are acted out are not their usual dreams. Patients describe them as being more vivid—horror dreams, dreams that are action-filled. They are battling with strange animals or unfamiliar characters, although, as with the NREM parasomnias, they too often mistake their bed partner for the threat.

In fact, cases are beginning to be reported of patients who have an overlap of both NREM and REM parasomnias, with sleepwalking, sleep terrors and RBD all occurring in the same person. In these cases, the patients' histories show a progression from a NREM parasomnia at a young age, to a later REM parasomnia, followed still later by a diagnosis of a neurodegenerative problem, most often Parkinson disease.

And as if that news were not troubling enough, RBD is strongly associated with another neurological sleep disorder, narcolepsy. This presents us with one of the classic dilemmas of science: When it comes to categorizing sleep disorders, are we better off as "lumpers" or "splitters"? Do we gain a better understanding of these disorders by finding their common features, or by finding what differentiates them from one other, and also from those who sleep well? I prefer a safe middle-of-the-road position, as I believe each approach can help us in understanding what has gone wrong.

Narcolepsy has happily had a recent major breakthrough that has increased our understanding of its pathology. It is one of the exceptions to the rule that sleep disorders occur only during sleep, leaving waking time relatively free of specific symptoms. Those with sleep apnea for the most part breathe without difficulty while awake; sleepwalking, sleep terrors, and nightmares by definition are confined to sleep. This is not so for those with narcolepsy, who are subject to episodes of complete or partial sudden loss of muscle tone while wide awake. These are known as attacks of *cataplexy*, and are triggered by some strong emotion. Sudden laughter, anger, surprise—even sexual excitement can leave these people limp enough that their knees buckle and they collapse and fall. If the attack is mild, perhaps just their chins sag, or they drop what they were holding. Those with narcolepsy also experience abrupt short episodes of sleep intruding into their waking lives. Although these may only last a few seconds or minutes, they can be frequent and dangerous if they occur while driving. These patients also have insomnia complaints, difficulties both staying awake and staying asleep. What is more, their transitions into sleep may be accompanied by instant dreaming (hypnagogic hallucinations), as can their morning awakenings (hypnopompic hallucinations). These dreams can seem very realistic. Further, narcoleptic patients may wake up but find they cannot move, as the atonia (lack of muscle tone) of their last REM period of the night persists for a few minutes into waking. All the features of REM sleep (dreams, loss of muscle tone, episodes of sleep) can intrude into waking and into NREM sleep. In other words, these individuals have difficulty with keeping their three major states of waking, NREM, and REM, separate. Narcolepsy is a disease characterized by a weak spot of another type—in the firmness of the boundaries between the usual physiological and psychological cyclical states.

To test for a diagnosis of narcolepsy, sleep clinicians conduct both a night of sleep testing using the standard PSG test, followed by a series of five opportunities to nap next day. This is called the *multiple sleep latency test* (MSLT). At night we expect to see a rapid onset of sleep, with REM sleep occurring close to sleep onset. We also see many periods of awakening within the night. The period before the first REM is much shorter than we noted in major depression. In patients suffering from narcolepsy, REM may begin after 5–15 minutes of sleep; in contrast in major depression REM is more likely to appear after 30–60 minutes. The second part of the sleep diagnostic testing, the series of naps the day after the night sleep test, will support the diagnosis if they too, show REM sleep intrusions into at least two out of five 20-minute opportunities to sleep, spread out at 2-hour intervals during the day. We also expect to see that, after having had a night of sleep as documented in the lab, these patients will fall asleep very quickly whenever they are given the chance to nap next day. It might take a normal sleeper about 15 minutes to fall asleep after having a full night's sleep, but a narcoleptic patient can do it in less than 5, and keep on doing it whenever we turn out the lights for another nap.

Genetic studies have looked into the coexistence of narcolepsy and RBD. These occur together in 25% of RBD patients. Human leukocyte antigen (HLA) testing by a blood draw demonstrates that these two disorders have at least one strong genetic similarity. What is common in their clinical presentation is the absence of muscle atonia in REM sleep, allowing dream enactment to take place in RBD. At the same time, the link between strong emotion and a sudden loss of muscle tone in waking (the cataplexy attack) blocks physical action by those with narcolepsy when it might be most necessary.

Much remains to be done to untangle the complex interactions of what started out as a simple "three states of being" model of the 24-hour cycle—waking, sleep, and dreaming—when sleep research first began. Now we see that there are boundary problems of many different kinds, and that when features normally confined to a certain part of the daily cycle overlap into others, the result is a variety of symptom pictures.

Next, I will turn to what has been the most neglected concept in modern psychology, that of the unconscious. As this term is often burdened with

Freudian baggage, some investigators prefer a more neutral one: nonconscious. Whatever we call it, nonconscious functioning is now enjoying a revival of interest and renewed experimental studies into its role in waking decision-making. I will put this together with what we have learned so far about the ongoing, nonconscious mental activity of sleep to further develop the model of the twenty-four hour mind at work.

Dreaming and the Unconscious | 9

Day unto day uttereth speech and
night unto night shewth knowledge.

—Psalms 19:1

Freud did not invent the concept of an unconscious mind, but he was its most successful salesman. The influence of his work on the popular culture of our time has been enormous. Our novels, songs, movies, plays, comic strips, and dance have all been deeply influenced by his ideas. Freud's conviction that our everyday behavior is influenced by unconscious impulses has shaped our thinking in unexpected ways. The jury decision in the Scott Falater trial is a case in point. When reporters asked for the reason behind the guilty verdict—for a crime for which no motive could be established—some stated that the decision was based on the belief that "he must have had unconscious hostility toward his wife." This shows how pervasive is our thinking about the power of the unconscious to influence behavior.

Our language, too, now includes many terms originated by Freud, such as the infamous "Oedipus complex," and concepts such as the id, ego, and super-ego are in common use. Entrenched is the belief that experiences in early child-hood are responsible for the balance of power among these basic elements of personality, an idea which is still invoked to explain our later self-defeating neuroses. If the superego is too strict, over-controlling the id impulses, a person will be so moralistic that he or she will be unable to enjoy life; and if the super-ego is too weak, a person will be under-controlled, impulsive, and act out.

Clinicians practicing "talk therapies" were those most strongly influenced by Freud's (and his daughter Anna's) theories of unconscious impulses and the ego's defenses, especially during the first half of the twentieth century. They strove to bring the early childhood unconscious learning histories of their patients into consciousness, so that their behaviors could be controlled by their rational adult minds. A successful treatment would ensure that the patient, although he may continue to do dumb things, would at least do them by choice rather than by unknowing compulsion.

Academic psychologists were skeptical of the colorful language of psycho-analytic theory and treated it as a set of untested and basically untestable hypotheses. Remember David Foulkes, who studied children's dreams to test Freud's idea that these would reveal the unconscious primitive wishes lurking below the surface in a sweet, innocent-looking child? Foulkes found no evi-dence supporting this theory in the dreams that young children reported. Although his conclusion was put in some doubt because his method required children to give a verbal report when awakened during sleep, it did reinforce the academic view that Freud's theory did not hold up to rigorous testing. Mostly psychologists of the 1950s were working hard to establish their profes-sion as a science, which meant putting an emphasis on hard data, those that were observable, measurable, and testable. That ruled out murky terms such as "mind" and "unconscious." These were considered too soft to meet the tests of verifiability. Freud was treated as an important historical figure, but students were discouraged from adopting psychoanalytic assumptions to explain behavior.

Two major contributions of the psychoanalytic theory of how adult person-ality develops, however, survived the trend toward strict behaviorism that began to take over psychology at this time. The first was the idea that behavior was the product of an ongoing dynamic interaction between basic physiologi-cal drives like hunger, which when gratified results in positive feelings of satis-faction, and the learned restraints on these drives required for social living, like manners. The social rules, when followed too strictly, were said to result in limitations on behavior and negative feelings of unhappiness and frustration. According to Freud, this over-control was a major problem for his patients.

The other surviving concept was Freud's emphasis on the importance of early developmental history, or how we acquired our understanding of society's rules as children. For most of us, this is a history largely forgotten, or at least not stored in an accessible form, and so unavailable for review. Who, after all, remembers how they learned not to talk about certain body parts or their functions in social situations? But Freud argued that these early learnings persist and may be in need of conscious revision.

Freud found that the best avenue for getting at this history was to create a context, in the therapy hour, in which the usual social constraints were reduced so that patients were free to wander mentally, to "free associate" and so reveal the mental maps they operate from without directed awareness. Freud went even further in exploring his own psyche, as well as those of his patients, by investigating what would happen when social constraints were eliminated altogether, when the moral monitors were off-duty—that is, when patients were alone and asleep. In sleep, these early primitive "wishes" (as Freud called them), which have been denied expression, emerge from memory and appear as dream images. The expression of these wishes in dreams, he posited, allowed otherwise forbidden impulses to be partially gratified through hallucinations and through our acceptance of them as "real" at the time. This mechanism was deemed a healthy one, as it keeps the peace. We are safe to express unsavory drives during sleep because we are unable to act them out.

Famously, Freud stated his position that "the interpretation of dreams is the royal road to knowledge of the unconscious activities of the mind." To that I reply with a quote from another famous author, "Aye, there's the rub." Shakespeare's Hamlet was uncertain how his dreams would help him resolve his difficult decision—whether to suppress his aggression or to act on his impulse to take revenge for his father's murder. Who is to say what a dream means? An interpretation that fits a theory is not the same as proof, which requires independent verification. Over the more than a century since the publication of Freud's *The Interpretation of Dreams*, many have tried to introduce objectivity into the study of dreams, treating them as data that can meet the tests of science and thus increase our "knowledge of the unconscious . . . mind." This effort has not received much recognition in the community of science, nor is the quest usually seen to be a worthy one. There are a few notable exceptions: Francis Crick, Jonathon Winson, Eric Kandel, Gerald Endelman, and Antonio Damasio have recognized that not all thinking is conscious, and that the brain holds the keys to understanding the complex infinite capabilities of the mind. These are some mighty big names, including some Nobel laureates. None is a sleep research scientist, although Crick did write a notable theory paper on dreaming. But each has pushed to expand our conception of the "mind" beyond the reductionism so characteristic of early behaviorists. As argued by these estimable scientists, we must use two methods to advance knowledge—we must look at what happens at the level of the synapses and in gene expression, and also how these findings support our understanding of ourselves and our world. Although each of these scientists has given a nod toward dreaming as a universal human experience, with the exception of Winson, none has gone so far as to support the investigation of dreams as basic to furthering our conception of the mind as a whole. In my view, there is much room for further exploration into the interactions of the mental activity of sleep and waking, of the conscious and the unconscious.

Science of the Unconscious

The opening up of the sleeping mind's activity through research into dreams took a long time to make any headway in the academic world. Today, even mental health clinicians have thrown out the idea that patients need to understand the past in order to correct their present unhealthy behaviors. They stay "in the moment," to help their patients take charge of their dysfunctional thinking and poor choices among behavior options. Cognitive behavioral therapy (CBT), the psychological treatment developed by Aaron Beck, has become the primary therapeutic method taught in U.S. graduate programs to clinical psychologists. Cognitive behavioral therapy requires patients to change negative thoughts directly without looking into their emotional roots. That means there is no need to make the unconscious conscious in order to revise a patient's dysfunctional assumptions.

Yet, the concept of the unconscious and the problem of explaining consciousness have continued to tease philosophers and neuroscientists alike. Philosophers argued and neuroscientists searched for methods more objective than Rorschach inkblots to access thought processes they could not observe directly—but still recognized as important to understand. Brain imaging technology, although it has advanced our descriptive understanding of the brain, does not reveal what is meant by the term *mind*. Brain imaging is useful for describing differences between groups, but identifying which parts of the brain are more or less active at a particular time does not tell us much about *how* they work. As that technology has moved to a more dynamic mode, using functional MRI (fMRI), we have become better able to watch the brain at work on various tasks—but only during waking.

Meanwhile, psychologists in other countries, not as bound by the limitations that American researchers place on what questions are thought to be scientifically respectable, have forged ahead, investigating the contribution of unconscious processes to human thinking, feeling, and acting. This work culminated in a recent important article, "A Theory of Unconscious Thought," written by a pair of social psychologists in the Netherlands, Ab Dijksterhuis and Loren Nordgren. The paper draws on their experiments comparing the efficacy of decisions based on conscious versus unconscious thinking. Dijksterhuis and Nordgren theorize that there are two distinct thought processes—the conscious and the unconscious—and they hypothesize on the circumstances under which each is the more effective and appropriate method for use in decision making. The idea itself is not new, but the support for it is.

A few American researchers have also been interested in subtle cognitive processes like "trusting our instincts," "insight," "empathy," "gut feelings," and "person perception." Some of this work was summarized and popularized in the book by Malcolm Gladwell, *Blink: The Power of Thinking Without Thinking*. Gladwell pulled together and described, entertainingly, work that has been ongoing in separate laboratories for a long time. He described the research of Paul Ekman on reading facial expressions, now being used for training airport screeners, and John Gottman's studies of the subtle communication patterns characteristic of good and bad marital interactions. Gladwell recognizes the power of what he calls the "adaptive unconscious," which holds much information that guides us to make decisions faster and often more correctly than our slower, more deliberative conscious thinking.

In contrast to the unconscious thought theory paper by Dijksterhuis and Nordgren, a second recent major position article was published in the same journal, written by a group of 19 authors, all well-funded and highly respected American research psychologists from the most prestigious universities in this country. In "Social Neuroscience: Progress and Implications for Mental Health," the message is that we need to transcend the departmental discipline-based boundaries of biological, neurological, and social sciences to create a multidisciplinary understanding of how we humans behave when we are successful and healthy. Further, they propose to apply this knowledge to preventing and treating those behavioral difficulties we recognize as mental disorders. The article reviews how brain imaging work relates to behavior and to social processes, and concludes with a call for "respecting the mutual influences of biological and social factors in determining behavior." This is a good mission statement, but not a word is written about unconscious processes or the need to look into the influence of the night mind on waking behavior.

One problem, in my view, is that those who study the waking mind seem to be unaware of the work of those who investigate the mind in sleep. A profound disconnect exists between these two approaches to knowledge. I expect that part of the difficulty lies in our being unable to point to a specific location in the brain as the home of what Freud would call the id, where the basic unconscious impulses reside. Even Gladwell distinguishes between what Freud meant by the

unconscious as a "murky place full of desires, memories, and fantasies too disturbing for us to think about consciously" and the sanitized version, in Gladwell's
words, of a "giant computer quickly and quietly processing a lot of data." Where
in the brain *is* the unconscious, for goodness sake?

That within the brain there is ongoing unconscious information processing
we can certainly agree—and that it can be pretty smart, too. But the unconscious seems to operate under different rules than does the mind we voluntarily
direct. The innovative work of Dijksterhuis and Nordgren's group in the
Netherlands on waking decision making is a good start toward better understanding of the unconscious. They compare the choices made when a person
arrives at a decision after attending to a problem, concentrating on the facts, to
those made when there is a delay before the choice is made. During this delay,
some participants were asked to focus on a different problem—a distracter.
Those who were distracted made better choices (at least under the circumstances of the experiments). Thus, the researchers' conclusion is that decision
making goes on "unconsciously" because of the limited capacity of the conscious mind when attention is directed elsewhere.

In the Dijksterhuis and Nordgren experiment that has received the most
attention, participants were asked to choose the best among four possible apartments, each with 12 different features. One apartment was made more desirable
with more positive features (it was bigger, had a friendly landlord); one was
made more undesirable with more negative features, and two were neutral,
with an equal number of positive and negative features. One group of subjects
had to make their choice among the four apartments immediately, another was
given 3 minutes to think over their options, and the last group was given 3 minutes to respond, but was also given a different task to complete during that
interval—a distracter. Then they were asked to make their apartment choices.
Attending to the alternate problem for that short time blocked the third group's
conscious thinking about which apartment was the best choice. In both groups
allowed a delay before making their choice, a mental process had been set in
motion and continued; participants knew they would be asked later to decide
which apartment was best for them. Those who shifted their attention to
another task actually chose the apartment with more good features more often.
The reason, Dijksterhuis and Nordgren suggest, is that these persons benefited
from the broader range of possibilities and consequences that were brought to
mind while their conscious attention was focused elsewhere, on a different task.
In contrast, the decision choices made by those who focused their attention
narrowly on the information before them were less successful at fulfilling their
own needs by their deliberate conscious thinking.

Although we may tell our children "turn off the music, you cannot concentrate on your homework when you are distracted like that," it seems that paying strict attention when working on a choice problem may not always be the wisest course. Turning attention away from a task often leads to a more insightful answer. We have phrases to describe processes like that—"I had a gut feeling," or "It just came to me in a flash." But we have really very little idea as to how this insight phenomenon works. One clear difference between the conscious and unconscious thought process in the apartment choice example is the role of attention. In one case, attention was focused narrowly on the problem, and in the other attention was shifted to another task; nevertheless a wider thought process is believed to continue, sub rosa, to search for the best choice. Where does this come from? Before we get too far into generalizing from this simple experiment, the authors remind us that conscious thought cannot take place without unconscious processes being active at the same time, all the time. Take talking, for example; words come and grammar rules are followed (usually) without any conscious effort on the part of the speaker. The bottom line is that conscious thought is constrained by low capacity; despite our attempts to multitask, we can only handle thinking very clearly about one thing at a time (consider the number of car crashes that occur while drivers are text messaging). That means we use only a subset of information during conscious thought and are guided by what is handiest—our habitual learned expectancies and organizing schemas. We are prone to jump to conclusions that confirm our expectations rapidly. Unconscious thinking is slower, it integrates more information. It is divergent in nature, and so may come up with new, unexpected ideas, whereas conscious thought is convergent and so more suited to "simple issues." Or, so say the authors of the unconscious thought theory article. Note a discrepancy here; Gladwell writes that the unconscious works quickly and the conscious mind is slower, whereas Dijksterhuis and Nordgren demonstrate the opposite about the speed of reaching decisions. Are they talking about different types of choices?

Usefulness of Dreams

What about sleep? When I discussed the studies demonstrating changes in mood from depression to mental health, I was examining how the mind works when the problem to be solved is not an experimental exercise, with limited time to produce an answer, but the need to adapt to a major life change—in this case divorce from a first marriage. This adaptation usually takes many months.

The persons involved in our studies were not students working for course credit but those for whom the problem is multifaceted and, for some, emotionally overwhelming. They were free, in sleep, to work on their emotional adaptation to this change without waking distractions. Our studies showed that some did this more effectively than others. Some felt better in the morning than they had before sleep, and after a few months proved to be no longer depressed. The important mental activity going on in the dream scenarios of these participants revealed the difference between those who did and did not remit from depression without treatment: it was their unconscious work on adapting to this major change by expressing emotions and linking images of the departing spouse to other memory material.

However, we found the immediate overnight positive mood change occurred in both those who recovered in the long run and those who did not. The difference was whether the better mood was sustained during the waking interval, not for 3 minutes, but for 12 or more hours—an entire day—before the next night of sleep. When the improved mood was sustained, as demonstrated by the scores on the next night's pre-sleep mood test (the Profile of Mood States [POMS]), and this was repeated at each testing point over the 5 months of the study, these people exhibited a return to mental health at the end of the study.

Although those who did and those who did not recover were diagnosed as equally depressed when they first joined the study, when I looked into why some lost the immediate benefit of a better morning mood following a night of sleep and reverted to being depressed during the intervening day, I found real differences in their dreams of the former partner. Those who remained depressed failed to link images from the present to older memories associated with their feelings about the marriage, failed to express their emotional response to the real change in their lives, and were not engaged or active in their own dream story. These blunted dreams were ineffective in changing the basic negative assumptions that continued to color their waking perceptions and responses to new experience. These are people who, one might say, cannot "take a compliment" because of their pessimistic worldviews.

Productive unconscious thinking, either in waking (as in the apartment choice experiment) or in sleep (as in the divorce study) does not always take place automatically. The active brain state in rapid eye movement (REM) sleep alone cannot guarantee a positive change in our minds; we also need access to an appropriate database of memories. These may be absent, or access to them may be blocked by other processes. This may account for the poverty of dreams in severe major depression. This was suggested by Eric Nofzinger, whose brain imaging studies of depressed and healthy controls while in REM sleep showed both groups had increased activity in the emotional brain areas known as the limbic system, but that the depressed also showed heightened activity in areas associated with higher executive functions not seen in the REM scans of healthy controls. Nofzinger theorizes that this might be what Freud would call the work of the "censor"; that this overactivity in the decision-making areas may be interfering with dream construction in those who are severely depressed.

For now, we can consider the term "unconscious" to be shorthand for a psychological process going on 24 hours a day, continuously relating present to past experiences and filing these into long-term memory. The selection of new experiences favors those that are emotionally toned. This process operates outside our voluntary direction and can be seen in its purest form in the mental content of REM sleep. I will offer an example of this in the next chapter, but first I will turn to studies that investigate whether sleep is active in selecting and storing new learning.

Sleep and Learning

A very early landmark psychology experiment conducted on two volunteers in 1924 showed that sleep contributes to preserving new learning better than a matched amount of waking time. Unfortunately, this work fell out of favor when its positive results (on learning nonsense syllables) could not be replicated with other kinds of materials. When sleep research began in earnest in the late 1950s, there were again some studies investigating problem solving over-night. The aim was to validate the many anecdotes that had sprung up in pop culture about breakthroughs of insight into vexing problems upon awakening. These studies were designed very much like the decision studies by the Netherlands team, except that they used a longer time delay than the 3 minutes. The delay was for a half or a full night of the usual 7 hours of lab-monitored sleep.

I conducted one of these studies in 1974, testing whether a period of sleep rich in REM time would yield different kinds of solutions (and more right answers) to unsolved problems than did a matched amount of waking time. Would REM sleep help people resolve some types of problems more effectively?

I chose three types of tasks for 24 students to work on. The materials were crossword puzzles, the Remote Association Test (RAT), and the Thematic Apperception Test (TAT). I wanted to test what difference the condition of waking versus an equal period rich in REM sleep would have on constructive mental work, and whether this differed depending on the type of problem involved. Since crossword puzzles have only one right answer for each clue, performance was expected to favor the waking condition. The RAT requires that subjects think "out of the box" to find one word that links three other very different words, making an unusual connection between them. For example, a word that links "snow," "base," and "costume" is "ball." These can get difficult, so performance on this test was predicted to favor the wider associations available in a sleep interval rich in dreaming. The TAT picture problem was designed to compare solutions to emotional interpersonal dilemmas, for which there is no one right answer. Participants were shown two cards taken from the TAT test. One card pictured a child looking at a violin, and the other depicted a well-dressed adult man standing beside an elderly woman who has her back turned to him. Each card was accompanied by a prepared "problem story." Those taking part were asked to write a dramatic "ending" to the story illustrated by each picture.

The students were given 10 minutes to work on each problem type (which was not enough to complete the task) before being stopped and told they would have 10 more minutes to work on the problems later. All had two different 3.5-hour intervals before their second chance to complete the task—one in regular daytime waking, the other in sleep. They worked on one type of task at a time over 3 days and 3 sleeping nights in the lab.

To ensure that the interval of sleep would have a high proportion of dreaming, the participants slept in the laboratory for the standard 7 hours of overnight recording time. However, during the first 3.5 hours, we prevented them from having REM sleep by waking them at the first signs that this stage of sleep was beginning. Ordinarily, the amount of REM sleep in the first half of the night is low, but this REM-deprivation awakening technique forced more REM time to rebound and increase in the second half of the night. For the sleep condition, participants were given the tasks to work on when they were awakened halfway through the night. After their 10 minutes of effort on the task of the night, they were allowed to go back to sleep for 3.5 hours without interruption. In the morning, they were asked to work for another 10 minutes on completing the problems they had started during the night.

The bottom line was that there was no difference between the number of additional correct solutions following an interval of waking and those following the sleep condition heavy with REM sleep. Both conditions yielded more right answers on the crossword puzzles and on the RAT tests. There was, however, a significant difference in the kind of story endings offered to the TAT pictures under the two conditions. After the REM condition, the story solutions the subjects constructed were surprisingly different from those they wrote after an equal waking interval. The waking story solutions were more often of the stereotyped happy ending type. We called them "Hollywood endings." After sleep, which included an average of 38% REM time, the solutions were more idiosyncratic. To some extent they were more "realistic" in that they took into account that the "main" character might not get their way and might have to compromise with other people's wishes.

There are several possible explanations for this result. One possibility is that the REM-depriving awakenings in the first half of the night were sufficiently unpleasant to bias the mood throughout the second half of the night and that this may have influenced the next morning story solutions to be more negative but realistic outcomes. Another possibility is that aborting REM sleep in the first half of the night interfered with the normal sequence of down-regulating the emotional tone of the dreams across the night (from more negative in the first dreams to more positive at the end of the night). By suppressing REM in the first half of the night, the normal within-sleep mood regulatory function of dreaming was blocked temporarily, making the dreams in the second half of the night the dreamers' first of the night, and so perhaps more negative. Thus, the dreamers would perhaps wake without the full resolution of negative mood following this manipulation. This might influence the story solutions away from the easy, clichéd happy ending they produced after a daytime waking period.

In any case, it was clear from this experiment that sleep accompanied by a large amount of dream time provided different associations and possibilities than did an equal waking period of time, but only with certain types of problems. More nuanced ideas were offered as solutions to emotional problems after sleep, ones that, had they been considered during the waking interval, would likely have been rejected. It seemed that dreaming opened up options that might make for more thoughtful solutions to emotional problems. This study raised more questions than it answered, but it did support the hypothesis that a period of time restricted to unconscious thought might lead to more complex considerations in response to emotional problems than would an equal period of waking time with an unknown mix of conscious and unconscious thinking.

When the studies on unconscious decision-making were published by the team in the Netherlands, others took up the challenge to try to replicate their findings. Scientists tested the effects of unconscious thinking using the distraction method that involved longer delays than the original 3 minutes, but did not test the effects of sleep.

By this time, the research results using animals were compelling in support of the benefit of sleep over waking in consolidating new learning. To study what the brain is doing to preserve new learning in long-term memory, microelectrodes were inserted into single cells in the hippocampi of rats (not exactly a technique that an American IRB committee is likely to approve for human volunteers). The most exciting finding was that the specific "place" cells in the hippocampus that are activated when an awake rat explores a new maze show the same activation pattern when the rat goes into slow wave sleep (SWS). This was proof that new learning is being retained by "reactivation" during sleep.

Investigators in Germany doing human studies then began to look into the contribution of sleep to performance on various memory tasks. They manipulated the amounts and stages of sleep in comparison to similar waking periods, testing their participants on declarative memory problems, words, facts, and spatial information, because these depended on an intact hippocampus. One of these studies attracted a good deal of media attention, as its finding was intriguing. Published in 2004, that study, called "Sleep Inspires Insight," established a few important points. First, insight into the solution to a mathematical puzzle occurs faster after sleep than after waking—but it also depends on the problem being practiced—but not solved—before sleep. Twice as many participants who had slept following attempts at solving the puzzle caught on to the solution when they woke up than did those who tried to solve it after an equal amount of time awake. This inspired research testing the benefit of the first half of the night, which is mostly SWS, versus the benefit of the second half of the night's sleep, which is largely REM sleep. We saw in my own study discussed earlier that REM-rich sleep did not have any advantage over waking for solving cross-word puzzles or RAT items, but perhaps was helpful in working out emotional problems by allowing participants to consider wider emotional associations. I may have missed the chance to see a positive effect on the less emotional problems by not testing the solutions following the first half of the night when SWS dominates.

Reactivation in the Human Brain

In the meantime, another breakthrough study published in 2008 got around the barriers to recording from single cells in the hippocampus of humans. An Israeli and American team was able to test the memories of a group of patients suffering from severe epilepsy. It is legitimate to implant microelectrodes into the brains of these patients, with their consent, as this technique is used prior to brain surgery to relieve their seizures. Brain mapping in this way helps to locate the site of the seizure problem and so avoid unnecessary removal of tissue important for functioning. These patients were awake during the tests of their memories. They were shown short film clips of popular TV shows, as well as more neutral scenes while the activity of single brain cells was being recorded. After a short distraction period, the patients were asked to think about what they had seen and to report what came to mind. Their responses, "I was remembering the Seinfeld film," for example, was accompanied by an identical match in brain cell activity while the person was recalling the film to the pattern recorded when that film was initially shown. Not all the film clips lit up the particular cells being recorded, so it is not clear whether the patients were less interested in some, not attending, or if the cells chosen to implant were not the right ones to catch those responding.

This was the first study to show reactivation of the same neurons basic to forming a new memory in humans while they were calling up that memory. Although the study did not capture the whole circuitry involved, it did confirm the thinking that we, just like rats, select experiences to be saved in memory by reactivating the original excitation response. This is an important step, but it leaves a lot still to discover.

If the mind is truly working continuously, during all 24 hours of the day, it is not in its conscious mode during the time spent asleep. That time belongs to the unconscious. In waking, the two types of cognition, conscious and unconscious, are working sometimes in parallel, but also often interacting. They may alternate, depending on our focus of attention and the presence of an explicit goal. If we get bored or sleepy, we can slip into a third mode of thought, daydreaming. These thoughts can be recalled when we return to conscious thinking, which is not generally true of unconscious cognition unless we are caught in the act in the sleep lab. This third in-between state is variously called the preconscious or subconscious, and has been studied in a few investigations of what is going on in the mind during the transition before sleep onset. David Foulkes designed a way to get at this thinking by telling the volunteers for a sleep study that he needed to test the equipment to make sure it was recording well before turning the lights out for sleep. He then left them to drift along with whatever spontaneous mental activity came to their minds, but if their recordings showed they were about to fall asleep, he interrupted and asked them to tell him what was going on in their minds at the time. He reported mostly random thoughts but also some pretty bizarre images. I have also used this method to catch what may be the subject of later dreams, and it is similar to Stickgold's work at trying to catch images occurring at sleep onset. This tracking of the mind across time is the theme of the next chapter, the roundup of mental activity in its various modes throughout the 24-hour cycle.

It is time for those who teach new research psychologists to wake up to the importance of what goes on in the dark of night, to grasp how the styles of thought that Freud named preconscious and unconscious interweave during the several stages of sleep, and to address the many questions remaining. How do these stages contribute to waking psychological behavior? What is it about sleep that is helpful in preserving some newly learned material?

What determines the paths of memory associations? Where and how does the erasing of memories deemed not important to maintain take place? There is so much for innovative researchers to do in order to close the gap between sleep research and the study of the mind awake. Readers take heed: Follow the science news. Researchers take heart: Cute data are awaiting.

The Role of Dreams in the | 10
Twenty-four Hour Mind: Regulating
Emotion and Updating the Self

Dreams are true while they last, and do we not live in
dreams?

—Alfred Lord Tennyson, *The Higher Pantheism*

Throughout this book, I have emphasized several themes that I want to tie
together now in this final chapter. The first is, as the title states, that the
mind is continuously active, although in different modes of expression, during
the two major alternating states of waking and sleep. (A shorthand way of cap-
turing this difference is to say metaphorically that we speak prose while awake
and poetry in sleep.) In addition, these two modes operate using different proportions of information from internal and external sources; in waking, there is
a wider lens open to receive and respond more to the external world, while in
sleep we are mostly confined to a narrower base of internal information both
new and old. The activity of the mind in these two modes serves different functions, although with some overlap. These functions are collaborative and interdependent in carrying out the job of using our wits to guide our behavior, to
keep us on track toward meeting our short- and long-term goals. We do this by
constructing models of the world we live in that allow us to anticipate events.
These models must be at least somewhat successful in their fit with reality, or we

get into various kinds of trouble. We call these models "schemas," and I have emphasized that they are continuously being modified from experience (by learning and retaining what we learn to apply in new situations). Taken together, the central schema is organized into what I have been calling the self-concept, our personal unique identity. The role of dreaming in maintaining this organization has been endorsed by one of the pioneers in sleep research, Michel Jouvet. In his book *The Paradox of Sleep: The Story of Dreaming*, he speculates about dream function: "Periodic dreaming would permit the repeated programming of unconscious reactions that are the basis of personality and individual differences in behavior."

The second theme I have developed is the role of emotion in influencing the smooth carrying out of the collaboration of the waking and sleeping mind. In waking, more of our conscious attention is directed toward monitoring the facts of the immediate and constantly changing external reality; in contrast in sleep, there is selective reactivation of some of the new waking experiences, with preference given to those that carry an emotional kick. This wake–sleep partnership continues to sort and store these emotion-related bits into networks holding similar previous experience. Under normal circumstances, when the waking level of emotion evoked the previous day is not extreme and there are similar experiences already stored, and if the night is one with adequate amounts and quality of sleep, this process results in the maintenance of the organizing schemas that keep our emotional well-being updated and in balance. Being in balance means that negative emotion is down-regulated over night, so that the next day begins with a calmer frame of mind with which to face the waking world. When a schema does not fit reality, when the predictions based on it fail to anticipate new events or misinterpret the responses of others, anxiety is generated. This has a disruptive impact on the quality and quantity of sleep, as we saw when we examined the impact of insomnia on both physical and mental health. In particular, when poor sleep persists, there is an increased likelihood of changes in the timing of rapid eye movement (REM) sleep and disturbances in the content of the dreams, as spelled out when we examined clinical depression.

The importance of the contribution of the sleeping mind to what and how new learning is retained, and how emotion affects this normal function, is now gaining wider attention and changing the paradigms for research. Those who previously restricted their studies of memory and decision making to time awake have begun to investigate the differences in performance when the experimental tasks—learning a new language for example—are followed by time awake, compared to equal sleep time. A few have begun to tease apart the role of emotion in how well memory tasks are performed by comparing sleep and wake time effects on memory when the tasks are chosen to be neutral (nonemotional) versus chosen to evoke negative feelings.

That there is a need for this work is a point made forcefully by Antonio Damasio in the Preface to his newly reissued book, *Descartes' Error*: "As the sciences of mind and brain flourished in the twentieth century . . . neuroscience gave a resolute cold shoulder to emotion research." Later he writes, "Emotion is finally being given the due that our illustrious forerunners would have wished it to receive, albeit a century late." Damasio's hypothesis, based on his scrupulous studies of patients with brain injuries that led to defects in decision making and a disorder of emotion, was that the participation of emotion in the reasoning process might be either "advantageous or nefarious depending both on the circumstances of the decision and the past history of the decider." His point is that emotion and reasoning continuously influence each other unless there is specific damage to the brain in the frontal area. This is a long way from earlier conceptions of academic psychology, which saw reason and emotion as separate topics of inquiry and located in separate neural systems.

We have looked at some of the new wave of work on decision making when the participants are given equal time in waking or time to sleep on it, as we examined the differences between conscious and unconscious modes of thinking. These studies produced mixed results until it was recognized that emotion was a wild card contributing to the effects researchers were finding. Remember Stickgold's studies of the carryover into sleep of learning to master the Tetris and Alpine Racer games? It was those who had a crash while skiing or some other emotionally toned memory who reported seeing these newly learned images when they fell into the first few minutes of sleep. These stimuli were of no relevance to those who had no previous experience; they did not carry over images from the study, but continued experiencing matters of their own concern in their transition into sleep.

A good deal of my work has been directed toward exploring whether the sleeping mind contributes to resolving waking emotional turmoil stirred up by some real anxiety-inducing circumstance. My method for these studies has been more "naturalistic" than experimental, as I chose to work with a life event that is often (but not always) associated with a major disruption of the schemas that organize waking experience. There are advantages and disadvantages to working with real events in a longitudinal format, the horizontal method across time. Although these studies follow research design principles, with hypotheses tested and the inclusion of matched control groups, I could not control what happened during the months between when the volunteers returned to have additional data collected. Divorce is one of those events that can be hard on emotional equilibrium—it is the emotional equal of pulling a chair out from under someone. Being dumped onto the floor requires adaptation to a new reality in order to pick oneself up and function again. This takes time—time to make major, lasting changes in emotional organizational schemas. Most research studies using experimentally induced emotional states involve very short-term time frames, hours rather than months. Those who took part in the divorce studies were involved in a multifaceted event affecting many areas of their lives. Students tested in laboratory-based studies were able to leave the problem behind once their participation in the experiment was over—my participants could not. In this way, I consider my studies are closer to reality—but they were less tidy than the experimental studies. Nonetheless, both strategies have furthered our understanding of the mind at work when in the predominantly conscious compared to the unconscious mode, and scientists who have used these different strategies are now approaching some integrative consensus.

For example, a 2008 study led by Harvard researcher Jessica Payne compared memory consolidation over two equally short waking intervals at different times of day to two long 12-hour periods—one over waking, the other containing the usual amount of sleep—in groups exposed very briefly to neutral or negative emotion-arousing pictures. The study showed that both short and long amounts of time spent awake led participants to forget both the negative foreground image of a car crash and the neutral background of the same picture. However, those whose 12-hour interval contained sleep, selectively recalled the negative emotion-arousing foreground image—but not the neutral background. Payne and her colleagues concluded that "sleep plays an active role in the consolidation of emotional memories," and that "sleep selectively consolidates those aspects of memory that are of greatest value to the organism." This was not the only recent study to show that sleep helps to consolidate memories of negative stimuli, but it was the first to show that sleep selectively preserves just the emotion-evoking image and does not offer an advantage over time spent awake for recall of nonemotional neutral features. High time, say I.

An even newer study reported in 2009 begins, "It is often hypothesized that sleep plays an emotional regulatory role. However, this putative normalizing function of sleep has received remarkably little empirical study." I am delighted to see work being done on this topic, especially as it suggests that findings using normal human participants may one day be applied to the treatment of post-traumatic stress disorder (PTSD) and other anxiety disorders. This study, led by Edward Pace-Schott, another Harvard scientist, found that sleep has a function, not shared by waking, of spreading the effect of psychological treatment directed toward reducing a fear response to one stimulus *to other similar stimuli*. Despite my necessary oversimplification of that study here, it is important to note its implications. The authors conclude that sleep is an important mechanism that will allow a daytime treatment, such as exposure therapy for fear-based disorders like phobias, to be effective in reducing a fear response to *other* related fear-inducing stimuli—which were *not* the primary target of the therapy—*but only if good sleep follows treatment sessions.* This means that good sleep hygiene measures, like a steady schedule of 7 or 8 hours, should be an essential component of any mental health treatment protocol where the aim is to reduce excessive fear responses. These patients typically have disturbed sleep, so they have less opportunity for the emotional learning gained from therapy during waking to be passed along in non-REM (NREM) and then on to REM sleep—the process by which it can be integrated into the network of related memories. Hot dog! I might even dub this "cute data." Finally, the study brings home the importance of coordinating the research on learning in both waking and sleep and of applying these findings to the treatment of emotional disorders that affect both daytime and nighttime functioning.

Although this work is a big step toward providing evidence of the interaction of sleep/wake psychological functioning, there has not yet been an effort to examine what exactly is going on psychologically during sleep that in this case enables the uncoupling of a learned fear response from a whole class of related waking stimuli. Pace-Schott and his collaborators are content to leave this as an unknown, a "black box," for now, except to recommend that therapy interventions take place as close as possible to sleep onset. This is to minimize the time awake before sleep has a chance to do its healthful linking or unlinking work.

As this work is pointing to a specialized psychological function of sleep in relation to negative emotions, does the night mind reveal a different organizational schema or self-conception from the one we are consciously aware of during the day? This is another theme of this book. This is, of course, familiar from Freud's reasoning that dreams allow the therapist to gain access to different data; namely, the forgotten memories from the early childhood training that he believed were the source of unhealthy adult personality patterns. His theory was based on the idea that the patient could not report this experience because it was held out of consciousness, but that this needed to be slowly and carefully brought under control of the conscious mind. This process would free the patient of the burden of keeping up the mental barrier that constrained the basic drives, particularly those of sex and aggression, and so would allow these to be expressed in more mature, gratifying behaviors.

There has not been much formal research designed to test this theory, apart from David Foulkes' study of children's dreams. We noted that Foulkes concluded that his results were not supportive of any difference between the waking cognition of the normal children he studied extensively and their dreams. Snyder agreed with this conclusion, that the dreams of normal young adults were "credible descriptions of waking events" and not very "interesting." He reports the typical dream is: "a clear, coherent, and detailed account of a realistic situation involving the dreamer and other people caught up in very ordinary activities and preoccupations, and usually talking about them." Maybe that is true of those who have minimal psychological difficulties, but those who are suffering from some emotional disorder can show us a difference in the nature of the organized schema of the self-concept as revealed in their dreams.

I did collect some data of this kind in the divorce study, and will offer one example from the dreams of a depressed participant I will call Rick. Rick had a major difference between his conscious self-description, at least the one he shared with me on his initial interview, and the one revealed on his first dream collection night in the laboratory. After taking the history of his courtship and marriage and his description of what led to the break up, as I did with all participants, I next asked him to describe his partner. Once the participants were comfortable talking with me freely, I also asked them to describe themselves— the "Who are you?" question. I then sat back and waited, giving them 5 minutes to tell me how they saw themselves in their own words.

Rick's divorce was just recently granted. He was then 34, tall, slightly built, sad-looking in his rimless glasses and with the rumpled look of an over-aged graduate student. The tests he took as part of the screening for the study and the psychiatric interview classed him as moderately depressed. His response to the Who Are You question surprised me. It was much shorter than others, who often took full advantage of the 5 minutes to tell me a good deal about themselves. Rick mumbled only: "I am a talented, ambitious, self-centered, sexy writer." I waited; after a long pause, he said finally, "I've run out of words." That night, he had his first sleep study without any experimental interruption and showed the disturbed sleep of the depressed with an early REM period and very little slow wave sleep (SWS). The next night, he had five REM periods and recalled a dream from each one. We can now look for the characteristics of the dream self, what Snyder called the "all-important 'I'" in his dreams. These constructs, or dream dimensions, are dichotomous, with paired opposite connotations. As I review his dream reports, I look for whether he presents himself as "talented" or "not creative," "ambitious" or "lazy," "self-centered" or "concerned for others," "sexy" or "not so motivated," and "a writer" or "otherwise employed." Here are the five dreams:

1. "I was talking on a cell phone, trying to get the bank on the phone. I was parked in a limo-type thing. I wasn't going anywhere. Outside it was like Florida, an Everglades-type thing."

2. "I was at the Board of Trade watching trading going on in the pit from an observation booth."

3. "I was at the lakefront with my Mom, telling her I wanted to buy some lakefront property. I was trying to get her to go in on it with me. She was saying I ought to buy it and put a chair by the lake so she can watch the lake. It was cold and rocky, and I was getting ready to shake her down for the big investment."

4. "I was at a Stephen King movie. A monster man was chasing a woman and a woman was sitting at a cabin and looking out the screen door and a car goes by and flips over and becomes a monster thing that can do anything he wants to do or be whatever he wants to be. I was one of the actors in this movie, and I said 'Whew. Close call, man.'"

5. "An actor friend of mine was trying to talk me into understudying him. He was selling me the idea, telling me that I would make great money. I had stopped at a cafeteria to check out a pretty woman in a bathing suit but I couldn't find her, so I made a phone call and was talking to this guy, then he was just there, trying to talk me into being his understudy."

If all we knew of Rick was based only on these five dreams could we see some of the self characteristics he acknowledged when he described himself to me at the first interview? That description sounded a very positive note. He presented himself as being talented as a writer and with the ambition to get what he wanted (self-centered). In the dreams, he presents a more negative picture. In these, he is motivated to acquire money and sex but fails to achieve either. In the first dream, he tries a conventional route by calling a bank but he cannot get through and is stuck, not getting anywhere, although he has put on a good front by riding in a limo. He is alone and takes no action to ensure a solution. In the second dream, he watches how others make money through the stock market. Again he appears to be seeking a quick and easy way to a fortune. He again is on his own and passive, just watching. In the third dream, he tries to manipulate his mother to finance him in an underhanded way. He appears to wish for things beyond his means and shows himself to be "self-centered," but also there is a hint of uneasiness about what he is doing in describing his behavior in relation to his mother as a "shake down." In the fourth dream, he is actively working as an actor but it is a fantasy that verges on a dangerous consequence, releasing unrestrained power to do whatever he wants. He feels relieved to have escaped from turning into a "self-centered" "sexy" monster who chases women but stops short, perhaps because of the watchful eye of his mother. In the final dream of the night, he is being advised by a friend to be more realistic and accept a lesser goal. Again he demonstrates his "sexy" self-definition as he pursues a pretty woman but misses out on finding her.

In sum, Rick's dreams do portray him as being ambitious, self-centered, and sexy, in line with his waking self-description, but he is unsuccessful in the first three dreams, in which he has regressed to become passive and dependent as well as magical in his thinking. He does not display two of the other positive characteristics of his waking self-definition. There are no dreams in which he is a talented writer. Rick is, at this time, depressed and this has brought him to doubt his talent; his dreams show a fear that he will "flip out" and do wild and crazy self-indulgent things. When he joined the study, he was employed doing various odd jobs and was ashamed to tell me that his mother was contributing to his financial support. He had lost confidence in himself and lost his sex partner by the divorce. However, halfway through the night in the fourth and fifth dream, he begins to show a change. He is no longer stuck. He becomes more active in addressing his problem by realizing his "close call" of turning into an impulsive monster and seems about to become more realistic and consider a less ambitious work role offered by a friend.

On the basis of this look into his sleeping mind, I placed a bet that Rick would recover from the clinical depression over the course of the study, even though he did not meet all the prediction criteria I developed to apply to the initial dreams. (He did not dream of his former wife, unless she is the bathing beauty who got away, and his dreams are rather simple in structure, with less affect, and involve fewer characters than those we saw in the dreams of those going through divorce who successfully recovered from their depression.) However, recover he did. At his last interview, I saw he had made some remarkable changes in his waking life. He changed his name; perhaps to distance himself from the father who had abandoned him and his mother. He cleaned up his appearance, styled his hair, and showed up in a fashionable suit and a smile. He had joined a local theater group and completed manuscripts for two plays, one of which was being produced and to which he invited me and my husband to attend. I was happy to see the positive terms of his self-description become realized (he was now actually being the talented writer). It was not a great play, but it was well reviewed. Shortly after the play closed, he took his ambition on the road and moved to California. There he was hired on as one of a team of script writers for a TV series. There he also met the beautiful girl of his dreams and married her. I lost touch with Rick except for taking note of his continuing on-screen credits.

No doubt Rick had made a successful recovery from his immobilizing depression—but what role did his dreams play in this? He faced some negative aspects of his behavior in the exploitative ways he was relating to his mother and to attractive women, and he rejected the goal of obtaining things beyond his means. By the last dream, he considers doing humbler work as his path to success. The main discrepancy between Rick's waking and dreaming self-conceptions was the "talented writer" central to his waking mind, which was absent in his dreams. Without that organizing core concept, he faces the threat of disintegration and then expresses relief at the mid-point of this dream sequence by saying "close call," meaning he has looked at the monster within and escaped from being the self-indulgent, dependent, acting-out failure.

This interpretation is speculative and may well be questioned by those who are skeptical of dreams having any intrinsic meaning. However, the evidence of an active night mind is undeniable, as are the within-the-night changes in the dream sequence that relate to changes in waking behavior. Rick's dreamed self shifts toward taking the first steps of becoming self-sufficient and self-fulfilled.

Now we have touched on three of the themes of this book: (1) The mind is active in both waking and sleep, (2) emotionally toned waking experience has a priority for being reactivated in sleep and stored in memory, and (3) dreams display images representing the interaction of recent emotional experience and previously associated images. When sampled in sequence across the night, dreams display the progressive down-regulation of disturbing emotion. This process is responsible for instituting adjustments in the organizing schemas, so that these become more useful in promoting waking adaptation to changed circumstances. This function is most effective when waking negative emotion is within a moderate range, neither too little when no major change is needed, nor too overwhelming.

The most important determinant of the self-concept is not set in our biology. The contribution of heredity to our temperament—whether we are outgoing or shy, excitable or calm—has been studied intensively in pairs of identical twins who have been raised from birth in different environments. The results of these studies estimate that not more than 30% of their adolescent behavior is accounted for by their shared heredity. Much more powerful is the context in which they live, particularly the legacy of the interaction with the caregivers who transmit to them the rules of the game. These are accompanied by evaluations of what are the good and bad ways to behave. These early learnings are not the whole story but do have long-lasting effects. Jerome Kagan, a psychologist who has spent a lifetime observing the behavior of infants and children over time puts it this way in his book *An Argument for Mind*: "Nothing about human thought, feeling, and behavior can be understood without acknowledging that humans evaluate events, others, and themselves on a good–bad continuum and try to acquire the personal features they judge as praiseworthy." What is praiseworthy differs a good deal by culture and the values of those who transmit it to the young. The schemas they develop to judge themselves and others are then a nature–nurture combination.

The thoughts, feelings, and actions we judge to be *not* praiseworthy, as they generate negative feelings, are more likely to be displayed in dreams. Freud would certainly say this is so, and Rick's dreams can definitely be read that way. But that does not imply that these "bad" thoughts and impulses are necessarily inaccessible to consciousness; only that, if these are disturbing and unattended or underattended in waking, they will carry over into sleep. This is supported by much of the research I have already described and by Fred Snyder's finding that even within his normal young adults negative emotions were more frequent in dreams than positive by a 2:1 margin. The recent study by Jessica Payne summarized earlier reported that waking exposure to stimuli that evoke negative feelings are remembered following a long interval containing 7 hours of sleep, but not remembered after an equal amount of time awake.

The final theme to tackle of the new model of the mind's work is the big question: How are the flawed schemas changed to become more accurate and better serve our goals of health and happiness? Must the unconscious be made conscious by way of retrieving the early learnings that have not served us well? Freud believed and taught psychoanalytic therapists to find the roots of current emotional problems in the dreams, as only there were the basic drives in their unacceptable form able to escape the powerful threat of being acted upon.

Contemporary psychotherapists have not followed that advice. Earlier, I noted that Carl Rogers had no place in his client-centered therapy for dreams, and no need to inquire into the patient's past history. His dictum for those in training in this method was "follow the feelings." Aaron Beck, father of cognitive-behavioral therapy, focuses on attending to the dysfunctional attitudes and habits of thought, without seeing any need to uncover their origin. Both Rogers and Beck are committed to helping their patients by having them attend to their current thoughts and feelings; that will help them understand and so change themselves. For Rogers, this meant helping them become aware of their unarticulated feelings, which were, as he would say, "at the edge of their awareness." These are the fears that he could hear in the trembling voice while the patient verbalizes just the opposite. "I am going to stand up and tell him to stop messing up my life." It was the therapist's job to catch the underlying feeling and to help patients recognize it by articulating it for them. "It is pretty scary to think of telling your father off." For Beck, it was the automatic thoughts that accompany speech, that although unspoken and unattended, powerfully relate to the emotional meaning of their experience. In other words, both Rogers and Beck target the ongoing preconscious mental activity of waking, not the unconscious, that is necessary for change to take place. Thus, both their theory and training programs were built on the belief that patients can learn to attend to their dysfunctional ongoing ways of misinterpreting reality and, by practicing, to catch this at the time it is happening, become aware of it, and so change their behavior. Although Rogers highlights the emotional and Beck the cognitive aspects of this, the mental activity that accompanies speech does not require patients to remember their dreams in order to access their past learnings. All they need is available in the sub rosa here and now.

The subconscious is also ongoing during dreaming. Remember that Fred Snyder also remarked that, in addition to what is happening in the foreground of the dream, there is "a more or less continuous background of reflections and attitudes, as well as clear evidence at times of inferential thinking, deciding, feelings of volition and of course, emotion." This description of the background flow of mental activity in dreams closely resembles what Rogers and Beck have pinpointed as what their patients must attend to in order to change the schemas through which they distort their perceptions, thoughts and feelings.

Not only is the subconscious ongoing as background in dreams, it is also the mental activity in the reports collected when sleepers are awakened from NREM sleep. These samples differ from dreams, as many studies have confirmed. They are more thought-like than sensory, and lack the story-like structure of dreams. They also lack the hallucinatory quality of being thought of as really happening, and are less emotional. When asked what was going on in their minds just before they are awakened from NREM, sleepers will typically say, "I was thinking about . . . " or, "I was wondering if . . . ". These, I believe, are part of the continuous stream of current concerns that are always ongoing. The only exception is that they may be present but not retrievable in SWS, perhaps because sleepers are hard to awaken then and repeated attempts to wake them may drive out the memory of these fleeting thoughts. These are important in our 24-hour model because dreams after all only occupy about 20%–25% of sleep time. This leaves about 50% of sleep in NREM mental activity that is retrievable, occurring between the dreams. What role does this play in the scheme of things?

We now have all the pieces we need to put together our model of the mind, but before mapping this out, I want to recognize some questions that may be on the reader's mind. What about the unconscious: Has that no place now? I am not throwing out the concept of the unconscious. As you may remember from the chapters on the sleepwalkers and other parasomnias that arise from SWS, I have stated that these show the basic drives in their unsocialized form operating without awareness or cognitive control. In other words, they are straight from what Freud might call the id impulses, from deep in the unconscious. I will return to place this piece in the jigsaw puzzle shortly. Before completing that, I want to address another question. Are the therapies of Rogers and Beck not missing out on important information by ignoring dreams? Can dysfunctional behavior really change without digging down to expose the roots of mistaken assumptions, hurt feelings, unrecognized angers, or a pervasive sense of unworthiness? Let me answer that by sharing with you an early disturbing dream of my own and its importance to me in self-understanding. This dream has features that have persisted over many decades, although the emotional component is now very much reduced. Originally, it invoked strong fear. Let's see in what ways it is modified and why it still returns, as an example of why I and many others are fans of the ingenious theater of the night.

Changes in a Frightening Dream

Despite my unofficial title, Queen of Dreams, I am not a consistent dream diary keeper. Like most people who work, I jump quickly out of sleep, shutting off the alarm and opening my eyes to check the clock. Is it really 6:30 A.M. already? Both of these behaviors, the muscle activity of abrupt movement and orienting of vision to outside stimuli, are REM stoppers, and therefore make dreams difficult to recall. However, sometimes a dream is so emotion-filled it imposes itself on our waking memory. I have chosen an example of one of these from my childhood because Freud holds these are the inaccessible roots of personality—a premise challenged by contemporary therapists.

My best guess is that I first had this dream at age 6 or 7. This is the way I remember it:

> Someone knocked at our front door, a big, heavy, wooden
> one with no window to see who was on the other side. I had
> to reach up to turn the handle, and then found a stranger, a
> tall man dressed as a harlequin in a suit of many colors,
> wearing a black mask. I knew from this that he was a robber,
> a bad man trying by his colorful costume to fool me into
> thinking that he was good. I was frightened and ran upstairs
> to hide in the bathroom, the only room that locked. My two
> older sisters were coming down the stairs as I dashed by.
> They laughed at me, saying, "Never show you are frightened
> of bad men. What you must do is charm them." I felt
> ashamed that they were better able to handle the situation
> than I. They went on down the stairs to greet the visitor, but
> I stayed locked in the bathroom, alone and frightened.

My method of parsing a dream for its meaning is to look for the descriptive terms and their opposites—the dream dimensions (I described these in my work with a nightmare patient). These are the categories we use to describe and evaluate ourselves and others. These organizing structures, which operate mainly on automatic pilot without our awareness, are developed early in life. In my experience, they can be seen most clearly in dreams. Now, what are the dimensions of this early dream of mine? I look first for the descriptors of the dream self. In this dream I was: *small, young, female, perceptive, frightened, withdrawing, ashamed, isolated.*

Next, I look for the opposites of these qualities in the other dream characters: *big, older, male, deceptive, calm, approaching, self-confident, sociable.* Two other general dimensions relate to the physical–psychological setting: *open/ closed*, and *inside/outside.*

Now we can see the structure of this dream. Its structure is made up of a few paired concepts. *I am small; the man and the door are big. I am young; my sisters and the man older. I and my sisters are female; the stranger is male. I am perceptive; the man and my sisters are deceptive. I am frightened; the others are calm. I withdraw; my sisters approach. I am ashamed; they are self-confident. I am isolated; the others are sociable.*

With these paired concepts and the addition of the narrative links connecting them we see the dream's purpose. There are two plots. The first poses an emotional problem: how to protect the present self in the face of an outside challenge, to welcome something new. This can be stated as, "The safety of a small, young, perceptive girl is threatened by a big, older, deceptive male. She withdraws from the encounter by retreating further inside and locking out the threat." In this version, the problem is solved, in the short term, by maintaining the self-concept as a vulnerable, asexual little girl. But this leaves her isolated, frightened, and in a limited place. In the second plot, the older sisters offer an alternate solution, which can be phrased, "When you are older you will not fear deceptive men but approach and charm (out-smart) them." The sisters represent a new developmental step in response to my dream question, "What happens if I open up to what is outside?" In the dream, I recognize that I am not yet ready to do as my sisters do, although I see that staying where I am is not a comfortable solution.

Over the many years since the first time I remember having this dream, some of the same dream dimensions have appeared repeatedly, like beads in a memory chain, especially when I have had a real and disturbing emotional experience relating to powerful men. The harlequin figure survives as a dream character many decades after his debut, but now he makes only very rare appearances and in a more muted form. One such revival of him in a dream was set at an annual meeting of the Association of Professional Sleep Societies, my professional home:

> I was standing at the back of a packed auditorium. On stage, awards were being announced. The first was given to a

well-known and well-respected psychiatrist. The man at the
microphone read out a long list of the awardee's
accomplishments. This was roundly applauded, and he was
led forward by an assistant to receive a plaque and to have
his picture taken. This routine was repeated for a second
man. The third award was then announced and, to my
surprise, it was for me. This time the assistant, dressed in a
harlequin suit, began fooling around on stage in a clownish
manner, peering into the audience, pretending he could not
see me. He walked up the main aisle and looked right at me
but instead of leading me forward to the stage, he turned his
back and threw up his arms in a gesture to show he gave up.
The audience started to leave. I asked the person standing
next to me, "Why didn't he speak of my work?" and "Why
did he make a joke of it?"

Are there dream dimensions in this scenario similar to those in the first
harlequin dream? A couple of these are easy to spot: I was female, the harlequin
was male. I was on the outside, literally standing on the fringe, while the others
were insiders, on stage or seated with their backs to me. In both dreams, I did
not meet the challenge with any positive action, but in the later dream I did not
run away. The harlequin is not as feared in this dream as when he had the role
of a robber. He was still engaged in robbing me, now of professional recognition, and in both dreams he was thinly disguised, a bad man pretending to be
good. Emotionally, both dreams were disturbing enough to be remembered.
What had I learned over all those years about managing my response to deceptive men?

On the positive side, even as a youngster I gave myself credit for seeing
through the deceptive guise of the bad man (his black mask gave him away). He
did not fool me, even though I was not old enough to know how to cope with
him; I ran. In the adult dream, I stood my ground and spoke of my feelings with
another person. This time, the bad man did not frighten me; the feeling was of
puzzled disappointment. I see him as only a "clown." Even more positively,
I knew in the later dream that I had produced a body of work that I deemed was
worthy of being noticed. The emotional message of that dream was: "You know
what you have done; you don't need the clowns to applaud you." Although not
wholly successful in eliminating the negative affect associated with not being
praiseworthy, this dream was not strong enough to initiate a major change in
the self-system.

I do not know what led to the first dream, but I am sure of the explanation for the later one. I had submitted a proposal to organize a symposium for the next annual meeting. It was turned down by the program committee. This was not the first rejection of a proposal I had experienced over the previous few years. Rationally, I knew that program time is limited and that there were many competing proposals; but emotionally I took this as a personal slight. The dream scenario is of being "overlooked" by a power-holder, one I saw as a deceptive clown pretending that withholding the prize was my own fault, due to my invisibility.

That explains what I dreamed, but not why. What was the function of that dream? I believe it was something like, "Your emotional reaction to rejection is due to your ambivalent feelings about being an outsider." In the original child-hood dream, in which I was frightened and retreated from the challenge of relating to an ambiguous male, the function was protective of the status quo, "I'm not ready to become socialized as a charmer." Knowing that I would have to make some adaptation to my self-system in order to interact with men in the future, I chose then (at age 6 going on 7) to take time to work this out on my own. In the adult version of the dream, a similar challenge is presented—modify the self-conception as an independent-minded sleep researcher if you want the reward of recognition as "one of the boys." In this dream, I replay the negative consequences of retaining the present self-concept. The emotional "problem" and its solution in both dreams are much the same, but as I became more self-confident professionally the dream affect (emotional load) was much reduced.

The reality rejection experience threatened a core characteristic of my self-concept—"I am a good sleep researcher who goes her own way." The nega-tive emotion associated with this experience reactivated in sleep the harlequin image. He is part of a network of older memories of challenges to a central self-definition: I am a smart little girl who figures things out for herself. In the adult dream, the challenge is to change my professional "independence," which I experienced as leaving me open to being ignored or robbed. That links the present threat to the image of a robber, a bad man pretending to be good and the old conflict between "go along or go it alone."

Would Freud agree that I have understood this emotional issue without the uncovering therapy? Probably not. He well might invoke the Oedipus complex and see the harlequin as representing my good/bad father and my mixed feel-ings when he would arrive on our doorstep after a long absence. However, I am content with the understanding I have reached, and it is now more of an amusing story than a threat.

Is dream interpretation necessary in order for change in a dysfunctional schema to take place? Uncovering the past may be helpful when some stubbornly troubling dreams persist—for instance those that shake us up and impose themselves on waking, like the PTSD nightmares. Perhaps some dreams have historical roots that should be examined in consciousness. Freud dismisses those who argue that there is no need to trace dreams to infantile wishes when recent experience is sufficient to account for their meaning; he chides such critics as missing the "latent" or hidden meaning of dreams. That kind of circular reasoning did not win Freud friends among scientists.

Freud faced a good deal of opposition when he first published *The Interpretation of Dreams*, some of which persists today. For example, there were then and still are contrary views about whether dreams serve to express important issues or just erase useless information from memory. A sophisticated recent hypothesis addresses this question. It comes not from human studies, but from research on the brain activity of rats. Italian scientist Antonio Giuditta and his colleagues call their proposal a "sequential hypothesis," which reconciles the conflict between Freud's view—that dreams illuminate early memories—and that of his critics, who held that dreams illustrate only what is being eliminated. The sequential hypothesis supports both functions. The memory clearing function is assigned to the slow-wave (delta) sleep that comes first in the sleep cycle, while the preservation and integration of novel material into preexisting memories is assigned to the REM sleep that follows. From their power spectral analysis of the electroencephalogram (EEG) brain waves of rats, the Giuditta group report that both memory clearing and memory retention are taking place during waking as well. They add that our older model, of three distinctive brain states—waking, NREM, and REM sleep, with distinctive functions for each—is too simplistic. While we are awake, some brain circuits are asleep (either in NREM or REM), and while asleep, either in SWS or in REM, some circuits may be awake or in lighter NREM. That confirms the concept of the permeability of the borders between states that I have speculated may account for the misperception of some insomniacs—that they have been awake all night, when in fact their sleep studies show they are having a mixture of light sleep and waking. It also accounts for the mixed condition characteristic of sleepwalker's behavior, which appears to be waking but is carried out without consciousness at the time and is not retrievable as a memory later. Brain waves during a sleepwalking episode show a slow progression from SWS to waking EEG activity. There are other data from human learning studies that support a sequential two-stage processing of new information to be held in memory during sleep, from NREM to REM.

Freud attempted to spell out the relation of the three streams of ongoing mental activity—the conscious, preconscious, and unconscious—and their contribution to the making and remembering of dreams. He used an analogy to explain this. "A daytime thought may very well play the part of an entrepreneur for a dream; but the entrepreneur, who as people say, has the idea and the initiative to carry it out, can do nothing without capital; he needs a capitalist who can afford the outlay, and the capitalist who provides the psychical outlay for the dream is invariably and indisputably, whatever may be the thoughts of the previous day, *a wish from the unconscious . . . an infantile one*" (italics in the original).

What data support, or fail to support this component of his dream theory? There are two assumptions to examine: The first is that dreams are expressions of unconscious drives, and the second is that these all spring from the infantile past. The day thoughts that carry forward into sleep are "neutral," and so allowed to make an appearance in dreams; but we should not be fooled by them. They are also smuggling contraband, forbidden messages from the untamed drives of the infant. Freud, borrowing the Oedipus myth from the Greeks, gave this idea universality. In short, all men have a buried impulse to slay their competitor, the father, and to take over as their mothers' sexual partner. Freud may have been right about his over-controlled Victorian patients, but today most troubling behaviors are the result of under- rather than over-control of basic drives.

There is now the evidence from the sleepwalkers that these drives are expressed when a failure of motor control allows us to observe the behavior that is performed after a SWS arousal. When we examined the NREM parasomnias, we saw many examples of sleepwalking actions that appear to be related to unsocialized drives of hunger (in the sleep eaters), of sex (in the sleep self-stimulators, interpersonal sleep sex behaviors or sleep sex), of aggression (in the sleep-related violence behaviors), of protection (in those who perform helping behaviors), and exploration (in those who wander into new territory). These indicate that drives, or motives, basic to our survival are active during deep sleep before REM when the first organized dream is formed. That these are unconscious behaviors is supported by sleepwalkers' failure to have awareness of what they are doing during an episode, and their continued puzzlement afterward. Also by these being behaviors unlike their waking personality.

Unfortunately, at this time, no studies have collected the REM dream reports of sleepwalkers, neither in children nor in adults. For the moment, let us assume that those with the underlying vulnerability to abnormal movement arousals out of the first NREM delta sleep, especially when they are sleep deprived, will display behavior relating to a basic drive. We would predict that if they had not arisen from bed but had been able to stay fully asleep, the REM period that followed would include images and a narrative related to that drive.

We would also expect that the emotions accompanying that narrative would be safely down-regulated by morning.

Summing Up Where We Stand on the Freudian Model

Freud made enormous contributions to our culture and to psychology as a field devoted to understanding human behavior. The first was his insistence that attention must be paid to the ongoing activity of the mind that is not conscious but that influences conscious perception and decision making in the waking state. The second was that the predominantly unconscious sleeping mind produces dreams, which are a data source for understanding the relation of present emotionally troublesome behaviors and the early learning of restraints of basic drives. Freud's theory, which rested a good deal on those two planks, was based on the recalled dreams of his patients and dreams of his own. This we know now to be a very limited and biased sample of the mental content of sleep.

At best, we are able to recall far fewer dreams from any night in comparison to what we can collect on a single night by making REM awakenings in the laboratory. Further, the dream recalled spontaneously is most likely to be the last one of the night, or one so disturbing it wakes us. Neither is a representative sample of all those experienced. The last dream is most often the longest, most bizarre, and most complex in structure, with scene shifts and time changes. It is also the most vivid in imagery and the most emotional. No wonder it takes a long time and much skill to decipher its meaning. It is also likely that any dream recalled later the next day (or even not until the next therapy session) will have undergone unpredictable changes from the original.

If we think of our mental activity as a flowing river, we can dip a bucket in and pull up a standard sample, say 5 minutes' worth, to examine its nature. Probably the simplest measure to apply to sleep thoughts is derived from the Foulkes Dream-like Quality of Fantasy (Df) scale. This scale ranges from 1 to 5, where 1 = no recall, 2 = a thought-like report, 3 = a single image, 4 = two or more images connected in a story-like structure, and 5 = a complex perceptual experience with a story-like structure, emotion, and belief that it is really happening. When the responses to the question, "What was going on in your mind just before I called you?" during awakenings from REM sleep are scored on this category system, normal sleepers average 3.8 for the REM reports of one night, with lower scores for reports of the first two REM periods and higher scores for reports drawn from the end of the night. Scores for reports collected from NREM awakenings are much more variable among normal sleepers, and even in normal sleepers tested at different times. There are those whose Df scores from NREM sleep stages are as high as their REM scores. These are known as NREM dreamers. There are far fewer of them than there are of those whose average scores from NREM sleep are low (between 1 and 2), who most often report "no recall," or give thought-like reports. This has resulted in a good deal of debate in the field. Since dreams can and do occur in sleep outside of REM periods, should we stop defining dreams on the basis of the neurophysiological characteristics of REM sleep altogether? That is a question still to be settled.

Non-REM dreaming then is another way in which people vary. The unique dream experience for most sleepers is tightly bound to the conditions of REM sleep, and this is the only condition in which this imagistic, unrealistic, story-telling occupies the spotlight of attention. There are others whose brain states are highly alert throughout all sleep. They are more likely to shift easily between preconscious and conscious styles even in waking and experience dream-like experiences in both REM and NREM sleep. Ernest Hartmann has described a personality difference that captures what I have been describing. He calls these *differences in the thickness of the boundaries of the mind.* There are those with thick and those with loose boundaries between reality and fantasy. The light sleepers, whose NREM sleep is sufficiently activated to sustain awareness of their mental activity, are ideal for tracking the progress of their waking concerns as they are recalled across the night.

Now we can illustrate these theoretical interactions in a diagram spanning the presleep waking hours and the 7 hours of sleep that follow, and finally the waking thoughts next morning (Fig 10.1). On a good night of sleep, good sleep-ers leave their conscious mind behind quickly, and this does not turn back on until they awaken some 7 or 8 hours later. During the first NREM cycle, some of the emotionally relevant experience that has been tagged as important during waking is now reactivated, and unimportant information is erased. If we are awakened during that first hour, we will report that we have been thinking, or musing, or wondering about something or other that has some emotional value

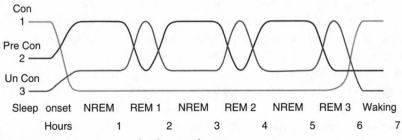

FIGURE 10.1 Cognition in wake/sleeping/dreaming

not fully recognized or resolved before falling asleep. In SWS, there is the added stimulus from one or more biological drives. After about an hour and a half, REM sleep begins. Along with the high brain activation of this sleep stage, there is an abrupt shift from loosely connected thoughts to a new format, with sensory images expressing one or more of the same emotion-related issues now energized as urgent concerns. Since the image-making mechanism has intersected with the preconscious thoughts, it will stimulate memories associated with those emotion-related thoughts that have been ongoing before sleep. Thus, a matching of new to older emotional memory material occurs in the first REM. After 10 or so minutes, this mental activity will give way again to the preconscious, which will take over the mind's eye, picking up and carrying forward some of the memory material from REM 1. That sequence is repeated until morning, when the last REM gives way to waking and the return of consciousness. As this now conscious state intersects with the complex blended memories of the last dream, as well as with some of the cognition taking place in the preconscious, it is no wonder we wake up saying, "I just had the craziest dream."

So, in good sleepers, the mind is continuously active, reviewing experience from yesterday, sorting which new information is relevant and important to save due to its emotional saliency. Dreams are not without sense, nor are they best understood to be expressions of infantile wishes. They are the result of the interconnectedness of new experience with that already stored in memory networks. But memory is never a precise duplicate of the original; instead, it is a continuing act of creation. Dream images are the product of that creation. They are formed by pattern recognition between some current emotionally valued experience matching the condensed representation of similarly toned memories. Networks of these become our familiar style of thinking, which gives our behavior continuity and us a coherent sense of who we are. Thus, dream dimensions are elements of the schemas, and both represent accumulated experience and serve to filter and evaluate the new day's input.

Sleep is a busy time, interweaving streams of thought with emotional values attached, as they fit or challenge the organizational structure that represents our identity. One function of all this action, I believe, is to regulate disturbing emotion in order to keep it from disrupting our sleep and subsequent waking functioning. In this book, I have offered some tests of that hypothesis by considering what happens to this process of down-regulation within the night when sleep is disordered in various ways.

First, we examined the emotional consequences when sleep is shortened over a period of more than 2 weeks, the definition of insomnia. The evidence is strong that short sleep, with frequent arousals, has a negative effect on mood.

Sleep loss also affects cognitive competency, impacting vigilance and the speed and accuracy with which we can learn new tasks. This too can lead to a change in our evaluation of ourselves. But perhaps the most important finding is that ongoing insomnia is for many a prelude to a diagnosis of major depression. If good sleep is generally followed by waking to a better mood, it is not surprising that lack of sleep or disrupted sleep has a negative effect on morning mood. This is true for rats as well as humans.

When major depression is severe, there is typically little or no deep SWS before an early onset of REM sleep. If deep sleep is where basic drives are activated, when there is no SWS, there will be little stimulation from these motives important for dream construction. No wonder the dream stories of the depressed are short, stark, flat in feeling, and feature a self character that is passive in the face of difficulties. If REM onset is very early, as it is when the depression is extreme, dream narratives may also not have the advantage of priming from reactivation of new information that normally takes place in the first NREM sleep. This is another reason why those seriously depressed are slow to change. In contrast, the dreams of those whose depression is moderate show progressively improving mood, from the beginning of the night to the end, and a more positive morning mood. This finding, which has been replicated now in several studies, confirms that dreaming has a mood regulatory effect when a waking negative mood is not extreme and the first REM does not begin so early that it precludes prior SWS. If the dream narratives include present waking concerns and link these to older memories, the balance of emotion shifts, from negative to positive within the night, instigating a corrective process, a change in the strategy of response to disruptive experiences. This may occur overnight or take many nights, depending on how pervasive is the waking depressive emotion and on the emotional tone of what has been filed in the memory networks.

Another sleep abnormality reviewed here was delayed dreaming due to an abnormal arousal from early SWS followed by nonconscious, nonrational behavior—including acts of overwhelming fear, aggression, exploration, feeding, or sexual behaviors. These demonstrate a breakdown of the mood-regulation function of dreams, when basic motivated behavior is enacted before it can be modulated by dreams that match these impulses to images of previous experiences.

Other sleep disorders reviewed—nightmares, PTSD, and REM behavior disorder—all share the symptom of REM sleep interrupted by fear or other strong negative emotions that appear as bad dreams. These wake the sleeper with full recall or lead to overt dream enactments. The inability of these sleepers to complete the dream cycle aborts the down-regulation of their negative emotions; as a result, these dreams are often repetitive, sometimes for years or even a lifetime.

The every-night sleep of the everyday person is not subject to as much disruption as in those we explored in the search for clues to the psychological functions of sleep. Often in science (especially science directed to understanding functions of the body), we learn about normal processes by studying what happens when those processes go wrong. When we examine the sleep and dreams of those who served as normal controls for our studies of depressed divorcing volunteers, those who were also going through a first divorce but without suffering from major depression, we can see the characteristics of sleep and dreams that work well in managing changes to the cognitive and emotional organizational schemas that guide behavior. The same characteristics are also observed in the dreams of healthy sleepers who are not experiencing any big change in their lives. That there is continuity of our mental lives across a 24-hour cycle, in which there is a normal distribution of waking, sleep, and dream proportions of time, is clear. The mind keeps working throughout the cycles of changes in brain activity, with only a hint of some "time off" in the deepest of SWS (Fig. 10.1).

There are many open questions still to be researched in order to fill out our understanding of ourselves as thinking, feeling, striving beings—in sickness and in health. What I have tried to do here is to lay out the evidence that mental activity is continuous; that sleep contributes to balancing our emotional lives by modulating the negative emotion invoked by those waking experiences that threaten the present organization of our self-structure. This process, continuously and creatively, overlays images of the new and older memories in REM sleep, threading them into new patterns that literally change our minds. These images may be hard to understand—not because they are forbidden, but because they are blends, more like complex paintings than linear texts. When all goes well, we wake refreshed and with a modified strategy for guiding our behavior toward fulfilling our now somewhat revised conception of ourselves. We are always works in progress. Dreams are a window onto the ongoing work of the mind during its essential night-shift.

Dreams Selected for | APPENDIX
Analysis from Scott
Falater's Dream Log

What follows is a selection of fourteen dreams from Scott Falater's log that include mention of his deceased wife, Yarmila.

1. September 13, 1999: "I have dreamt a lot about hiking or driving on arduous journeys up the sides of mountains or through strange cities. Sometimes I have been alone, other times my children have been with me. Sometimes we have been lost or stuck at an obstacle. Sometimes, Yarm, my wife, has been driving, but she always knew where we were going and would be encouraging me."

2. June 4, 2000: "I am standing on a railing about 6 feet up, looking down into a truck's bed, through a gap in its gate I can see the hindquarters of a *huge* deer. It's wearing shiny armor. An old guy and Yarm are going to pull the deer out using a rope tied to it like a leash. The old guy says the deer is dead but I see that it is bucking around in the truck. I warn them that they could be hurt. The old guy hands me an old single-action rifle with one bullet in it. I realize that I should shoot the deer if it becomes dangerous. I load the rifle, and they pull the deer out backwards. I am nervous because I have never shot a deer, and don't know where to hit it to kill it. I keep aiming at its chest and head and see the rest of the dream along the rifle's barrel. The deer breaks loose from Yarm and the old guy but it runs into the street, which is flooded with a foot of rapidly flowing water. There is some traffic in the street, and the deer runs to the far

side near an intersection and lays down on all fours in the water. Suddenly, its mate (a male) and son emerge from under water right in front of it where they had been hiding. All of us, including the deer, are happy to see the deer family reunited."

3. September 17, 2000: "Yarm and I have dinner at a restaurant. When we are done, we go out to the curb in front to look for a ride. It is a wet and sloppy Chicago-style winter day. We decide to walk and head up the street which turns into a forest trail. We walk for a while with one arm around each other's waists. I start out very happy but the deeper into the woods we go, the more troubled I become. Finally I stop us, hug Yarm and cry on her shoulder, that I love her and am going to miss her. She's confused and perplexed and asks me what I am talking about."

4. May 13, 2001: "I have started a new job that I am pleased about. It is my first day and I am getting oriented. My new boss is a cigar-chomping, hard-bitten guy who looks and talks like Charlton Heston. He's gruff and tough, but I like him. I get to my office and try to call home, but as I dial I realize that Yarm is gone and I don't have a home to call anymore."

5. September 18, 2002: "I'm lying on a sofa, totally relaxed, with my head in Yarm's lap. She is stroking my hair and speaking softly to me and gently caressing me, making me feel like I don't have a care in the world."

6. September 21, 2002: "I'm in Europe on business, and travel home the long way through Thailand. I arrive in America and find myself in snowy woods. I hear something of interest and go to the base of a snowy hill to check it out. People are there talking of an historical incident that happened there in which a guy preached mightily and founded a small now dead religion that's a variation of Mormonism. I'm not impressed, and I leave. Now I find myself in the company of an earnest, very pretty black-haired young woman who holds my hand. We are walking on a sidewalk in a wintry Midwestern suburb. I'm very protective of her as we cross streets, etc. I wonder why she is interested in me. She wants me to lead a revival of that religion. I really don't want to do it, saying 'I just did all that religion stuff in my life. That was enough.' I arrive alone at my mother's house. It's late at night and dark. I go through the dark rooms and find Yarm sitting on the couch waiting up for me. I am overwhelmed with relief and happiness. I sit next to her and we talk. It's late and time for us to go to bed. I'm totally energized. Megan and Mike appear as little kids in their pajamas and say they were afraid to sleep. I tell them that I am there to protect them and any monsters will have to get through me first. They laugh and run back to bed. I go in the dining room and the table is set for a birthday party for me which never happened because I was gone in Europe. I sense that Yarm is a little unhappy with me because of that. I find several packages on the table addressed

to me from Lisa, one of my prison pen-pals. I wonder how Yarm feels about that—whether she's jealous or not."

7. March 3, 2003: "I am in a nice, large department store, dealing with a nice salesman. I buy gift certificates from him, good for all new bed linens and quilts and matching window treatments for four bedrooms, which will cover my whole family. I worry a little that I am springing an unwelcome surprise on Yarm and she won't like it, but it is after all a gift for her anyway. I complete the transaction and the salesman motions vaguely toward the section where the merchandise will be that Yarm will choose from. I head that way and think about how I will spring this surprise on Yarm but then I run right into her. She's buying some jewelry for herself. She's dressed very nicely and is happy to see me. I wait with her until she is done and we walk together. I tell her about the gift, and we go to find the merchandise section but we can't find it. We find an information counter staffed by young women. We ask them where to go. They get rude and snippy. We strike out on our own. I feel very proud to have this fancy woman with me. We go down a staircase but it is all a parking garage full of cars. I go to turn around but Yarm goes up to some people and asks if this is the parking garage. I get frustrated and yell, 'Of course it is, now come on.' We start scaling the stairs but now there are lots of iron bars and obstacles in the way. I climb through them easily but Yarm has turned into a 2- or 3-foot tall dwarf with a huge shaved head. She gets ahead of me climbing through the obstacles, like a kid on the monkey bars. I feel badly that I am responsible for her new condition and hope that it isn't permanent."

8. October 17, 2004: "I am riding a large octagonal elevator up. It's one that has appeared in previous dreams and it scares me because it is unreliable. I ride it up to the top of a tall corporate building and am supposed to get back on it. All eight doors go up like garage doors opening up the whole top floor. But the elevator floor is unstable and tippy. I refuse to get on when it tips downward under my weight. The president of the company gets impatient with me and muscles the floor back to be level. In a flash Yarm and I are in the basement of the building. It's a multilevel parking structure. We stand on a balcony on the uppermost level and see signs designating which cars go on which levels, Volvos, Caddies, etc. The setting is industrial with exposed pipes. Yarm nimbly climbs down some pipes nearby to the floor on the lowest level below. I try to follow but quickly get stranded, straddling a pipe with nothing to steady me. I freeze, afraid to fall, and then try to back up, but I make *very* slow progress. Yarm grows impatient, and I don't want to disappoint her."

9. September 12, 2005: "I am like a ghost or a leper, not part of reality. I see Yarm standing in line at an outdoor restaurant. I shadow her, and she knows I am there. We have been separated, and she has Megan living with her. Yarm fills

me in about what's happened since we have been apart. She speaks of a rich life of fun events and much happiness brought to her by a new man. I feel like shit. I say to her that she is in love with the new guy. Yarm hesitates but says she thinks she is. I feel worse. I look at her carefully, she looks great. She is dressed very well and has a glow about her. I touch her and tell her she should just get a divorce from me. My touch leaves mud on her coat. Yarm doesn't answer. Yarm is seated at a table on a column high up above the crowd and is served five plates of food all at once so she has a choice of what to eat. I watch her, and we talk as she picks at a plate. I know I am very unhappy, and Yarm at one point says 'It's been nice to see how the other half lives.' That again makes me feel like a failure. She gets up to leave. I tell her not to act like a stuck-up rich person, but Yarm picks up a full plate of food from the table, says something angry to the maitre d' and throws the food on the floor and leaves. A waitress slips on the food and sprains her ankle. I go to her aid, and we poor people commiserate about our mistreatment at the hands of the privileged."

10. September 16, 2005: "I am in a new SUV. Yarm is driving us through traffic. There is a huge storm battering us and there is heavy traffic, but Yarm drives crazily and angrily and dangerously. We are on our way to pick up the kids, so I try to say something to calm her down, but I don't feel worthy to lecture her in any way."

11. December 5, 2005: "I'm in a big messy house with lots of nooks and crannies and ornate furniture. Even though it's my house, I own nothing but my two handfuls of prison clothing. I see Yarm causally toss even these aside. I get angry and grab them up saying that surely there's room in this big place for my few things. I start going through drawers and shelves and see nowhere where my things can go."

12. December 5, 2005 (same night as above): "Yarm and I are in an SUV driving along a long, isolated, muddy road. I am very upset by something even though the vehicle is handling the sloppy conditions well enough. I get out of the car and go back the way we came on foot. I stop and look back. Yarm is still in the SUV but she hasn't started driving away. The scene is very lonely, and I feel sad and vindicated at the same time."

13. February 25, 2006: "I am at home alone, working hard to clean it up. The home is dark and dreary. Yarm comes home from work late. I'm a bit peeved with her. She suggests we go out to dinner. I agree reluctantly. We get in the car and head down the road. I am driving. She is unhappy with me, and I am pretty angry. She then says that she probably won't eat because she is not hungry. I then start making U-turns to go back home, saying that we were only going out because she wanted to. She is surprised at my anger, and I feel a bit like a jerk, but it feels good to let my anger out."

14. July 25, 2006: "I am with Yarm and have been released from prison. She wants sex badly, as I do. She is being dominant and orders me about in bed and that is perfectly fine with me. I'm just so thrilled to be with her again; except I cannot seem to satisfy her even when I do all the things that used to really get her going."

References

Introduction: References and Notes

Listed below are the two papers from Dr. Kleitman's lab that are mentioned as the start of the new era of sleep research with the discovery of rapid eye movement (REM)/dream sleep. The third is Kleitman's comprehensive book, updated with the new material from his lab as of 1963. In it, he quotes Edward Jacobson, another University of Chicago physiologist, who is noted for his work on the "relaxation response," the start of the modern practice of relaxation therapy. Dr. Kleitman states: "In his (Jacobson's) own words (1937), 'When a person dreams . . . most often his eyes are active. Watch the sleeper whose eyes move under closed lids. . . . Awaken him . . . and you are likely to find . . . that he had seen something in a dream'" (p. 94).

Good ideas are a matter of timing. They are often rediscovered over and over until they hit the right time to be noticed. Kleitman tips his hat to recognize Jacobson's prior insight into the eye movement and dreaming connection.

1. Aserinsky, E., and Kleitman, N. (1953). Regularly occurring periods of eye motility and concomitant phenomena, during sleep. *Science, 118*: 273–274.
2. Dement, W., and Kleitman, N. (1957). Cyclic variations in EEG during sleep and their relations to eye movements, body motility, and dreaming. *EEG and Clinical Neurophysiology, 9*: 673–690. Preliminary communication. *Federal Procedures, 14*: 37, 1955.

3. Kleitman, N. (1963). *Sleep and wakefulness*, revised and enlarged edition. Chicago: University of Chicago Press.

Chapter 1.   In the Beginning: The Early Days of Sleep Research

1. Freud, S. (1954). Project for a scientific psychology (1895). In: M. Bonaparte, A. Freud, and E. Kris (Eds.), *The origins of psychoanalysis: letters to Wilhelm Fliess* (pp. 347–445). English translation. New York: Basic Books.
2. Freud, S. (1955). *The interpretation of dreams* (1900). English edition. New York: Basic Books.
3. Dijksterhuis, A., and Nordgren, L. (2006). A theory of unconscious thought. *Perspectives on Psychological Science*, 1(2): 95–109. [This is the article which put the waking unconscious back on the agenda for psychologists to address.]
4. Kupfer, D. (1976). REM latency: a psychobiologic marker for primary depressive illness. *Biological Psychiatry*, 11: 159–174.
5. Cartwright, R.D. (1991). Dreams that work: the relation of dream incorporation to adaptation to stressful events. *Dreaming 1*: 3–9.
6. Rogers, C.R. (1951). *Client-centered therapy*. Boston: Houghton-Mifflin Co.
7. Rogers, C.R., and Dymond, R. (1954). *Psychotherapy and personality change*. Chicago: University of Chicago Press.
8. Cartwright, R.D. (1966). Dreams and drug induced fantasy: a comparative study. *Archives of General Psychiatry*, 15: 7–15.
9. Dement, W. (1960). Effect of dream deprivation. *Science*, 131: 1705–1707. [This is the study that showed REM is a robust system, not easily suppressed and will increase on the nights following suppression called REM rebound.]
10. Meier, C., Ruef, H., Ziegler, A., and Hall, C. (1968). Forgetting dreams in the laboratory. *Perceptual and Motor Skills*, 26: 551–557.
11. Hobson, J.A., and McCarley, R.W. (1977). The brain as a dream state generator: an activation-synthesis hypothesis of the dream process. *American Journal of Psychiatry*, 134: 1335–1348. [This is the paper that argued that dreams are not created in sleep but in our awakening association to random stimuli.]
12. Allison, T., and Van Twyver, H. (1970). The evolution of sleep. *Natural History*, 69: 58–65. [A charming history of how NREM and REM sleep developed over time in different species.]
13. Roffwarg, H., Muzio, J., and Dement, W. (1966). Ontogenetic development of the human sleep-wakefulness cycle. *Science*, 152: 604–619. [This paper suggests that the function of the high rate of active sleep in the embryo and infant is to stimulate neuronal growth and connections in the brain.]

Chapter 2.   Collecting Dreams: Watching the Sleeping Mind

1. Foulkes, D. (1982). *Children's dreams: longitudinal studies*. New York: John Wiley and Sons.

2. Snyder, F. (1970). The phenomenology of dreaming. In: L. Madow and L.H. Snow (Eds.), *The psychodynamic implications of the physiological studies on dreams* (pp. 124–151). Springfield IL: Charles C. Thomas.

3. Meier, C., Ruef, H., Ziegler, A., and Hall, C. (1968). Forgetting dreams in the laboratory. *Perceptual and Motor Skills, 26*: 551–557.

4. Weisz, R., and Foulkes, D. (1970). Home and laboratory dreams collected under uniform sampling conditions. *Psychophysiology, 6*: 588–596.

5. Lloyd, S., and Cartwright, R.D. (1995). The collection of home and laboratory dreams by means of an instrumental response technique. *Dreaming, 5*: 63–73.

6. Mamelak, A., and Hobson, A.J. (1989). Nightcap: a home based sleep monitoring system. *Sleep, 12*:157–166.

7. Nofzinger, E. (2005). Neuroimaging and sleep medicine. *Sleep Medicine Reviews 9*: 157–172. [This is a very good overview as an introduction to imaging findings with great illustrations and good references.]

8. Bassetti, C., Vella, S., Donati, F., Wielepp, P., and Weder, B. (2000). SPECT during sleepwalking. *Lancet, 356*: 1484–1485.

9. Monroe, L., Rechtschaffen, A., Foulkes, D., and Jensen J. (1965). Discriminability of REM and NREM reports. *Journal of Abnormal Psychology, 2*: 456–460. [This study shows the clear differences between reports from NREM and REM awakenings in the lab.]

10. Rasch, B., and Born, J. (2008). Reactivation and consolidation of memory during sleep. *Current Directions in Psychological Science, 17*: 188–192. [A very good short summary of where we are currently in understanding the relation of sleep to memory consolidation. Also contains a very good reference list.]

11. McNaughton, B., Barnes, C., Battaglia, F., Bower, M.R., Cowan, S., Ekstrom, A., Gerrard, J.L., Hoffman, K.L., Houston, F.P., Karten, Y., Lipa, P., Pennartz, C.M., and Sutherland, G.R. (2003). Off-line reprocessing of recent memory and its role in consolidation: a progress report. In: P. Maquet, C. Smith, and R. Stickgold (Eds.), *Sleep and brain plasticity* (pp. 225–246). New York: Oxford University Press.

12. Smith, C., and Lapp, L. (1991). Increases in the number of REMs and REM density following an intensive learning period. *Sleep, 14*: 325–330.

13. Smith, C., and Smith, D. (2003). Ingestion of alcohol just prior to sleep onset impairs memory for procedural but not declarative tasks. *Sleep, 26*: 185–191.

14. Stickgold, R. (2003). Memory, cognition and dreams. In: P. Maquet, C. Smith, and R. Stickgold (Eds.), *Sleep and brain plasticity* (pp. 17–39). Oxford: Oxford University Press.

15. Ambrosini, M.V., and Giuditta, A. (2001). Learning and sleep: the sequential hypothesis. *Sleep Medicine Reviews, 5*: 477–490.

Chapter 3. Short Sleep and Its Consequences: Insomnia

1. CDC, Centers for disease control and prevention. (2005). Percentage of adults who reported an average of ≤6 hours of sleep per 24 hour period by sex and age group, United States 1985–2004. *Morbidity and Mortality Weekly Report, 54*: 933.

2. National Sleep Foundation, Sleep in America Poll. (2005). Accessed at http://www .sleepfoundation.org/_content/hottopics/2005_summary_of_findings.pdf.

3. Rechtschaffen, A., Bergmann, B., Everson, C., Kushida, C., and Gilliland, M. (1989). Sleep deprivation in the rat: X. Integration and discussion of the findings. *Sleep, 12*: 68–87.

4. Monroe, L. (1967). Psychological and physiological differences between good and poor sleepers. *Journal of Abnormal Psychology, 72*: 255–264.

5. Dement, W. (1960). The effect of dream deprivation. *Science, 131*: 1705–1707.

6. Kripke, D., Garfinkel, L., Wingard, D., Klauber, M., and Marler, M. (2002). Mortality associated with sleep duration and insomnia. *Archives of General Psychiatry, 59*: 131–136.

7. Spiegel, K., Tasali, E., Penev, P., and Van Cauter, E. (1999). Impact of sleep debt on metabolic and endocrine function. *Lancet, 354*: 1435–1439.

8. Gottlieb, D., Punjabi, N., Newman, A., Resnick, H., Redline, S., Baldwin, C., and Nieto, F. (2005). Association of sleep time with diabetes mellitus and impaired glucose tolerance. *Archives of Internal Medicine, 165*: 863–867.

9. Van Dongen, H., Maislin, G., Mullington, J., and Dinges, D. (2003). The cumulative cost of additional wakefulness. Dose-response effects on neurobehavioral functions and sleep physiology from chronic sleep restriction and total sleep deprivation. *Sleep, 26*:117–126.

10. Dement, W. (1972). *Some must watch while some must sleep* (p. 64). San Francisco: W.H. Freeman and Co.

11. Ford, D., and Kamerow, D. (1989). Epidemiologic study of sleep disturbances and psychiatric disorders: an opportunity for prevention. *Journal of American Medical Association, 262*: 1479–1484.

12. Ayas, N., White, D., Manson, J., Stampfer, M., Speizer, F., Malhorta, A., and Hu, F.A. (2003). Prospective study of sleep duration and coronary heart disease in women. *Archives of Internal Medicine, 165*: 205–209.

13. Vioque, J., Torres, A., and Quiles, J. (2000). Time spent watching television, sleep duration and obesity in adults living in Valencia, Spain. *International Journal of Obesity and Related Metabolic Disorders, 24*; 1683–1688.

14. Smith, M., Perlis, M., Park, A., Smith, M.S., Pennington, J., Giles, D., and Buysse, D. (2002). Comparative meta-analysis of pharmacotherapy and behavior therapy for persistent insomnia. *American Journal of Psychiatry, 159*: 5–11.

Chapter 4. Sleep and Dreams in Depression

1. Perlis, M., Giles, D., Buysse, D., Tu, X., and Kupfer, D. (1997). Self-reported sleep disturbance as a prodromal symptom in recurrent depression. *Journal of Affective Disorders, 42*: 209–212.

2. Kupfer, D.J., and Foster, F.G. (1972). Interval between the onset of sleep and rapid eye movement sleep as an indicator of depression. *Lancet, 2*: 684–686.

3. Jarrett, D. B., Miewald, J., and Kupfer, D.J. (1990). Recurrent depression is associated with a persistent reduction in sleep-related growth hormone secretion. *Archives of General Psychiatry*, *47*: 113–118.

4. Armitage, R., Rochlen, A., Fitch, T., Trived, M., and Rush, J. (1995). Dream recall and major depression: a preliminary report. *Dreaming*, *5*: 189–198.

5. Barrett, D., and Loeffler, M. (1992). Comparison of dream content in depressed vs. non-depressed dreamers. *Psychological Reports*, *70*: 403–406.

6. Nofzinger, E., Mintun, M., Wiseman, M., Kupfer, D.J., and Moore, D. (1997). Forebrain activation in REM sleep: an FDG PET study. *Brain Research*, *770*: 192–201.

7. Giles, D., Kupfer, D.J., Rush, J.A., and Roffwarg, H. (1998). Controlled comparison of electrophysiological sleep in families of probands with unipolar depression. *American Journal of Psychiatry*, *155*: 192–199.

8. Vogel, G., Thurmond, A., Gibbons, P., Sloan, K., Boyd, M., and Walker, M. (1975). REM sleep reduction effects on depression syndromes. *Archives of General Psychiatry*, *32*: 765–777.

9. Vogel, G., McAbee, R., and Barker, K. (1977). Endogenous depression improvement and REM pressure. *Archives of General Psychiatry*, *33*: 96–97.

10. Clayton, P. (1986). Prevalence and course of affective disorders. In: A.J. Rush and K. Altschuler (Eds.), *Depression: brain mechanisms, diagnosis and treatment* (pp. 32–44). New York: Guilford Press.

11. Cartwright, R. (1983). Rapid eye movement sleep characteristics during and after mood disturbing events. *Archives of General Psychiatry*, *40*: 196–202.

12. Kramer, M. (1993). The selective mood regulatory function of dreaming: an update and revision. In: A. Moffitt, M. Kramer, and R. Hoffman (Eds.), *The functions of dreaming* (pp. 139–195). Albany, NY: The State University of New York Press.

13. Indursky, P., and Rotenburg V. (1998). Change of mood during sleep and REM sleep variables. *International Journal of Psychiatry in Clinical Practice*, *2*:47–51.

14. Cartwright, R., Young, M., Mercer, P., and Bears, M. (1998). The role of REM variables in the prediction of remission from depression. *Psychiatry Research*, *80*: 249–255.

15. Cartwright, R., Luten, A., Young, M., Mercer, P., and Bears, M. (1998). The role of REM sleep and dream affect in overnight mood regulation: a study of normals. *Psychiatry Research 81*: 1–8.

16. Cartwright, R., Baehr, E., Kirkby, J., Pandi-Permual, S.R., and Kabat, J. (2003). REM sleep reduction, mood regulation and remission from untreated depression. *Psychiatry Research*, *121*: 159–167.

17. Cartwright, R., Agargun, M., Kirkby, J., and Freidman, J. (2006). Relation of dreams to waking concerns. *Psychiatry Research*, *141*: 261–270.

Chapter 5. Sleepwalking into Danger: Murders Without Motives

1. Ohayon, M. (2000). Violence and sleep. *Sleep and Hypnosis*, *2*: 1–7.

2. Broughton, R. (1968) Sleep disorders: Disorders of arousal? *Science*, *159*: 1070–1078. [This is the landmark article that showed the NREM parasomnias had related sleep characteristics.]

3. Broughton, R. (2000). NREM parasomnias. In: M. Kryger, T. Roth, and W. Dement (Eds.), *Principles and practice of sleep medicine*, 3rd edition (pp. 693–706). New York: Saunders.

4. Bonkalo, A. (1974). Impulsive acts and confusional states during incomplete arousal from sleep: criminal and forensic implications. *Psychiatric Quarterly*, *48*: 400–408. [This is the definitional study of sleepwalking that results in a crime is a sleep disorder.]

5. American Psychiatric Association. (2000). *Diagnostic and statistical manual of mental disorders*, 4th edition, text revision (pp. 639–644). Washington DC: APA.

6. American Academy of Sleep Medicine. (2000). *The international classification of sleep disorders (revised): diagnostic and coding manual*. Westchester, IL: American Academy of Sleep Medicine.

7. Cartwright, R. (2000). Sleep-related violence: does the polysomnogram help establish the diagnosis? *Sleep Medicine*, *1*: 331–335.

8. Broughton, R., Billings, R., Cartwright, R., Doucette, D., Edmeads, J., Edwarth, M., Erwin, F., Orchard, B., and Turrall, G. (1994). Homicidal somnambulism: a case report. *Sleep*, *17*: 253–264. [This is the case report of the Ken Parks murder case.]

9. Cartwright, R. (2004). Sleepwalking violence: a sleep disorder, a legal dilemma and a psychological challenge. *American Journal of Psychiatry*, *161*: 1149–1158. [This is the report of the Scott Falater murder case.]

10. Schenck, C., and Mahowald, M. (1995). Polysomnographically documented somnambulism with long distance automobile driving and frequent nocturnal violence: parasomnia with continuing danger as a noninsane automatism. *Sleep*, *18*: 765–772.

11. Pilon, M., Montplaisir, J., and Zadra, A. (2008). Precipitating factors in somnambulism: impact of sleep deprivation and forced arousals. *Neurology*, *70*: 2284–2290. [This study shows the conditions for eliciting sleepwalking behavior in true sleepwalkers and not in controls in the laboratory.]

12. Lecendreux, M., Bassetti, C., Dauvilliers, Y., Mayer, G., Neidhart, E., and Tafti, M. (2002). HLA and genetic susceptibility to sleepwalking. *Molecular Psychiatry*, *8*: 114–117.

13. Bassetti, C., Vella, S., Donati, F., Weilepp, P., and Weder, B. (2000). SPECT during sleepwalking. *Lancet*, *356*: 484–485.

14. Gaudreau, H., Joncas, S., Zadra, A., and Montplaisir, J. (2000). Dynamics of slow-wave activity during NREM sleep of sleepwalkers and control subjects. *Sleep*, *23*: 1–6.

15. Espa, F., Ondze, B., Deglise, P., Billiard, M., and Besset, A. (2000). Sleep architecture, slow wave activity, and sleep spindles in adult patients with sleepwalking and sleep terrors. *Clinical Neurophysiology*, *111*: 929–939.

16. Guilleminault, C., Poyares, D., Abat, F., and Palombini, L. (2001). Sleep and wakefulness in somnambulism: a spectral analysis study. *Journal of Psychosomatic Research*, *51*: 411–416.

[References 14–16 are the three papers showing NREM parasomnias have a low delta activity from spectral analysis scoring. The difference between the conventional scoring of the percent of delta waves in each 30 seconds of sleep and the count of each wave that meets the criteria as being a delta wave is like the difference between analog and digital TV. Slow wave activity is a more precise measure.]

17. Mendelson, W. (1994). Sleepwalking associated with zolpidem. *Journal of Clinical Psychopharmacology*, *14*: 150. [This is the first report that zolpidem (Ambien) produces sleepwalking in the laboratory that is not produced by another sleep aid.]

18. Guilleminault, C., Palombini, L., Paleyo, R., and Chevrin, R. (2003). Sleepwalking and sleep terrors in pre-pubertal children: what triggers them? *Pediatrics*, *111*: 17–35.

Chapter 6.   More NREM Parasomnias: Those Who Injure Themselves, Seek Food or Sex, Explore and Protect

1. Schenck, C., Hurwitz, T., Bundlie, S., and Mahowald, M. (1991). Sleep-related eating disorders: heterogeneous syndrome distinct from daytime eating disorders. *Sleep*, *14*: 419–431.

2. Winkelman, J. (1998). Clinical and polysomnographic features of sleep related eating disorder. *Journal of Clinical Psychiatry*, *59*: 14–19.

3. Mangan, M. (2001). *Sleepsex: uncovered*. Accessed at Xlibris.com.9-103. [This is a compilation of sleep-sex cases based on telephone interviews about the experience. The author speculates about how this disorder affects relationships of men and women.]

4. Shapiro, C., Fedoroff, J., and Trajanovic, N. (1996). Sexual behavior in sleep: a newly described parasomnia. *Sleep Research*, *25*: 367.

5. Schneck, C., Arnulf, I., and Mahowald, M. (2007). Sleep and sex: what can go wrong? A review of the literature on sleep related disorders and abnormal sexual behaviors and experiences. *Sleep*, *30*: 683–702.

6. Schenck, C., and Mahowald, M. (1996). Long-term nightly benzodiazepine treatment of injurious parasomnias and other disorders of disrupted nocturnal sleep in 170 adults. *American Journal of Medicine*, *100*: 333–337. [This study reports a 12-year longitudinal study of the effects of nightly averaging 1.1 mg clonazepam to be effective in controlling both NREM and REM parasomnias without the development of tolerance.]

7. Hurwitz, T., Mahowald, M., Schenck, C., Schulter, J., and Bundlie, S. (1991). A retrospective outcome study and review of hypnosis as treatment of adults with sleep walking and sleep terror. *Journal of Nervous and Mental Disease*, *179*: 228–233.

8. Hauri, P., Silber, M., and Boeve, B. (2007). The treatment of parasomnias with hypnosis: a five-year follow-up study. *Journal of Clinical Sleep Medicine*, *3*: 369–373.

[These two papers (References 7 and 8) show a short-term hypnotic induction treatment is cost-effective in controlling sleepwalking and sleep terrors over a 5-year period in half the patients.]

9. Hirshkowitz, M., and Schmidt, M. (2005). Sleep-related erections: clinical perspectives and neural mechanisms. *Sleep Medicine Reviews, 9*: 311–329.

10. Hirshkowitz, M., Moore, C., and Karacan, I. (1992). Sleep-related erections during REM sleep rebound. *Sleep Research, 21*: 319.

11. Broughton, R. (1968). Sleep disorders: disorders of arousal? *Science, 159*: 1070–1078.

12. Schenck, C., Boyd, J.L., and Mahowald, M.W. (1997). A parasomnia overlap disorder involving sleepwalking, sleep terrors and REM sleep behavior disorder in 33 polysomnographically confirmed cases. *Sleep, 20*: 972–981.

Chapter 7. Sleepwalking and State of Mind in the Courtroom

1. Thomas, T. (1997). Sleepwalking disorder and *mens rea*: a review and case report. *Journal of Forensic Science, 42*: 17–24.

2. Espa, F., Dauvillers, Y., Ondaze, B., Billiard, M., and Besset, A. (2002). Arousal reactions in sleepwalking in adults: the role of respiratory events. *Sleep, 25*: 871–875. [This is the first controlled study to show esophageal pressure monitoring precipitates arousals in sleepwalkers but not in controls.]

3. Guilleminault, C., Palombini, L., Pelayo, R., and Chervin, R. (2003). Sleep walking and sleep terrors in prepubertal children: what triggers them? *Pediatrics, 111*: 17–25. [This is a well controlled study showing that subtle sleep disordered breathing (SDB) in children who present with sleepwalking and/or sleep terrors are often comorbid and will respond to a surgical treatment that controls the SDB.]

4. Lateef, O., Wyatt, J., and Cartwright, R. (2005). A case of Non-REM parasomnia that resolved with treatment of obstructive sleep apnea. *Chest, 28*: 461 S. [This is the Cat Killer case, showing treatment of the sleep apnea stopped the dangerous NREM parasomnia behaviors.]

5. Nofzinger, E., and. Wettstein, R. (1995). Homicidal behavior and sleep apnea: a case report and a medicolegal discussion. *Sleep, 18*: 776–782. [This is the report of The Prisoner who shot his wife and had severe sleep apnea.]

6. Ohayon, M., Guilleminault, C., and Priest, R. (1999). Night terrors, sleepwalking and confusional arousals in the general population, their frequency and relationship to other sleep and mental disorders. *Journal of Clinical Psychiatry, 60*: 268–276. [This is a further analysis of the data from the epidemiological study of almost 5,000 persons in the United Kingdom. The prevalence rates are based on self-report and so are thought to be an under-estimate by the authors. This makes the case that NREM parasomnias are not rare.]

7. Kales, A., Jacobson, A., Paulson, M., Kales, J., and Walter, R. (1966). Somnambulism: psychophysiological correlates. 1. All night EEG studies. *Archives of General Psychiatry, 14*: 586–594. [This is a lab study of four sleepwalker children and controls using the long cable to continue monitoring the electroencephalogram (EEG) during a sleepwalk. Children were induced to walk by standing them up in slow-wave sleep. Good illustrations of sleep recordings.]

8. Broughton, R. (1968). Sleep disorders: disorders of arousal? *Science, 159*: 1070–1078. [This is the classic definitional paper unifying the NREM parasomnias by their sleep stage and timing similarity.]

9. Joncas, S., Zadra, A., Paquet, J., and Montplaisir, J. (2002). The value of sleep deprivation as a diagnostic tool in adult sleepwalkers. *Neurology, 58*: 936–940. [This study showed 10 sleepwalkers by history had an increasing number of SWS arousals and these were of increased complexity on a recovery night following 36 hours of sleep deprivation. Matched controls had no episodes in either baseline or recovery nights.]

10. Pilon, M., Zadra, A., Adams, B., and Montplaisir, J. (2005). 25 hours of sleep deprivation increases the frequency of and complexity of somnambulistic episodes in adult sleepwalkers. *Sleep, 28:A* 257.

11. Pilon, M., Montplaisir, J., and Zadra, A. (2008). Precipitating factors in somnambulism: impact of sleep deprivation and forced arousals. *Neurology, 70*: 2284–2290. [This is the final paper in this series showing the discriminating power of fewer hours of sleep deprivation when combined with increasing auditory tones.]

12. Mahowald, M., and Schenck, C. (2004). Parasomnias: sleepwalking and the law. *Sleep Medicine Reviews, 4*: 321–339.

13. Cramer Bornemann, M., Mahowald, M., and Schenck, C. (2006). Parasomnias: clinical features and forensic implications. *Chest, 130*: 605–610.

14. Mahowald, M., Schenck, C., and Cramer-Bornemann, M. (2007). Finally: sleep science for the courtroom. *Sleep Medicine Reviews, 11*: 1–3.

15. Cramer Bornemann, M. (2008). Role of the expert witness in sleep-related violence trials: virtual mentor. *American Medical Association Journal of Ethics, 10*: 571–577.

16. Willis, C. (2008). The CHESS method of forensic opinion formulation striving to checkmate bias. *Journal of American Academy of Psychiatry and the Law, 36*: 535–540.

17. Fenwick, P. (1987). Somnambulism and the law: a review. *Behavioral Science and the Law, 5*: 343–357.

Chapter 8. Warnings from the Land of Nod: Nightmares and REM Behavior Disorder

1. Lavie, P., and Kaminer, H. (1991). Dreams that poison sleep: dreaming in holocaust survivors. *Dreaming, 1*: 11–21.

2. Ross, R., Ball, W., Dinges, D., Kribbs, N., Morrison, A., Silver, S., and Mulvaney, F. (1994). Rapid eye movement sleep disturbance in posttraumatic stress disorder. *Biological Psychiatry, 35*: 195–202.

3. Levin, R. (1994). Sleep and dreaming characteristics of frequent nightmare subjects in a university population. *Dreaming, 4*: 127–137.

4. Neilsen, T., and Levin, R. (2007). Nightmares: a new neurocognitive model. *Sleep Medicine Reviews, 11*: 295–310. [An excellent review and integrative model with a fine bibliography of historical and current references.]

5. Germain, A., and Neilsen, T. (2003). Sleep pathophysiology in PTSD and idiopathic nightmare sufferers. *Biological Psychiatry, 54*: 1092–1098.

6. Hublin, C., Kaprio, J., Partinen, M., and Koskenvuo, M. (1999). Nightmares: familial aggragation and association with psychiatric disorders in nationwide twin cohort. *American Journal of Medical Genetics, 88*: 329–336. [This study establishes a genetic basis for chronic nightmare vulnerability.]

7. Krakow, B., Hollifield, M., and Schrader, R. (2000). A controlled study of imagery rehearsal for chronic nightmares in sexual assault survivors with PTSD: a preliminary report. *Journal of Traumatic Stress, 13*: 589–609.

8. Lancee, J., Spoormaker, V., Krakow, B., and van den Bout, J. (2008). A systematic review of cognitive-behavioral treatment for nightmares: toward a well-established treatment. *Journal of Clinical Sleep Medicine, 4*: 475–480.

9. Miller, W., and DiPalato, M. (1983). Treatment of nightmares via relaxation and desensitization: a controlled evaluation. *Journal of Consulting and Clinical Psychology, 51*: 870–877.

10. Cartwright, R., and Lamberg, L. *Crisis dreaming: using your dreams to solve your problems* (pp. 105–113). New York: Harper Collins, 1992; San Francisco/San Jose: ASJA Press 2001 iUniverse, San Jose.

11. Mellman, T., Nolan, B., Hebding, J., Kulick-Bell, R., and Dominguez, R. (1997). A polysomnographic comparison of veterans with combat-related PTSD, depressed men and non-ill controls. *Sleep, 20*: 46–51.

12. Schenck, C., Bundlie, S., Patterson, A., and Mahowald, M. (1987). Rapid eye movement sleep behavior disorder: a treatable parasomnia affecting older adults. *Journal of the American Medical Association 257*: 1786–1789. [This is the first study defining a new parasomnia of REM sleep.]

13. Schenck, C., Boyd, J., and Mahowald, M. (1997). A parasomnia overlap disorder involving sleepwalking, sleep terrors, and REM behavior disorders in 33 polysomnographically confirmed cases. *Sleep, 20*: 972–981.

14. Schneck, C., and Mahowald, M. (2002). REM sleep behavior disorder: clinical, developmental, and neuroscience perspectives 16 years after its formal identification. *Sleep, 25*: 120–138.

15. Morrison, A., Sanford, L., Ball, W., Mann, G., and Ross, R. (1995). Stimulus-elicited behavior in rapid eye movement sleep without atonia. *Behavioral Neuroscience, 104*: 972–979.

16. Zagrodzika, J., Hedberg, C., Mann, G., and Morrison, A. (1998). Contrasting expressions of aggressive behavior released by lesions of the central nucleus of the amygdala during wakefulness and rapid eye movement sleep without atonia in cats. *Behavioral Neuroscience, 112*: 589–602.

17. Desseilles, M., Dang-Vu, T., Schabus, M., Sterpenich, V., Maquet, P., and Schwartz, S. (2008). Neuroimaging insights into the pathophysiology of sleep disorders. *Sleep, 31*: 777–794. [A good updating of brain imaging for many sleep disorders as well as the structural and functional abnormalities in RBD leading to dream-enactment.]

18. Khatami, R., Landolt, H-P., Achermann, P., Retey, J., Werth, E., Mathis, J., and Bassetti, C. (2007). Insufficient non-REM sleep intensity in narcolepsy-cataplexy. *Sleep, 30:* 980–989.

Chapter 9. Dreaming and the Unconscious

1. Crick, F., and Mitchison, G. (1983). The function of dream sleep. *Nature, 304:* 111–114. [This is the statement of the problem of the need for a "dreaming" mechanism for unlearning, or clearing space of useless new experience.]

2. Winson, J. (1985). *Brain and psyche: the biology of the unconscious.* New York: Anchor Press. [Winson bases his hypothesis of dream function on the finding of the three year period between memory retrieval requiring the hippocampus and long-term consolidation no longer needing a reactivation via the hippocampus to state "REM sleep is a process whereby the flow of recent events and past associations is tapped into and integrated into a guide for future behavior" (pp. 213). "These strategies for coping with the real world . . . constitute the *unconscious personality.* One feature of which is the "motivations underlying and guiding behavior" (pp. 229).

3. Kandel, E. (2006). *In search of memory: the emergence of a new science of the mind* (pp. 376–390, 429). New York: W.W. Norton. [Kandel comments on the problems of explaining consciousness and its relation to the unconscious mind and the problem of relating both to neural activation of brain structures.]

4. Etkin, A., Klemenhagen, J., Dudman, M., Rogen, R., Hen, E., Kandel, E., and Hirsch, J. (2004). Individual differences in trait anxiety predict the response of the basolateral amygdala to unconsciously processed fearful faces. *Neuron, 44:* 143–155. [This is the report of the study comparing brain imaging differences in response to human faces denoting fear when exposed with enough time for a conscious perception versus an exposure so rapid that the response was due to unconscious perception. Different areas of the amygdala are activated with the degree of response to unconscious recognition related to the subjects' level of trait anxiety.]

5. Endelman, G., and Tononi, G. (2000). *The universe of consciousness: how matter becomes imagination.* New York: Basic Books. [This is a brain model of consciousness that defines it as involving groups of neurons that are widely distributed and that engage in strong, rapid reentrant interactions. The authors introduce the concept of value systems that signal continuously the state of the organism and produce a sudden burst of activity whenever something important occurs. These select circuits are sufficiently similar to those previously adapted, which is the basis for the emergence of consciousness.]

6. Damasio, A. (2005). *Descartes' error: emotion, reason and the human brain.* New York: Penguin Books.

7. Dijksterhuis, A., and Nordgren, L. (2006). A theory of unconscious thought. *Perspectives on Psychological Science, 1:* 95–109.

8. Gladwell, M. (2005). *Blink: the power of thinking without thinking*. New York: Little Brown & Co.

9. Ekman, P. (1992). Facial expressions of emotions: new findings new questions. *Psychological Science*, 3: 34–38.

10. Gottman, J., Katz, L., and Hooven, C. (1997). *Meta-emotion: how families communicate emotionally*. Mahwah, NJ: Lawrence Erlbaum Associates.

11. Cacioppo, J., Amaral, D., Blanchard, J., Cameron, J., Carter, C.S., Crews, D., Fiske, S., Heatherton, T., Johnson, M., Kozak, M., Levenson, R., Lord, C., Miller Ochsner, K., Raichle, M., Shea, M.T., Taylor, S., Young, L., and Quinn, K. (2007). Social neuroscience: progress and implications for mental health. *Perspectives on Psychological Science*, 2: 99–123.

12. Cartwright, R., Baehr, E., Kirkby, J., Pandi-Perumal, S., and Kabot, J. (2003). REM sleep reduction, mood regulation and remission in untreated depression. *Psychiatry Research*, 121: 159–167.

13. Nofzinger, E. (2005). Neuroimaging and sleep medicine. *Sleep Medicine Reviews*, 9: 157–172.

14. Jenkins, J.G., and Dallenbach, K.M. (1924). Obliviscence during sleep and waking. *American Journal of Psychology*, 35: 605–612.

15. Cartwright, R. (1974). Problem solving: waking and dreaming. *Journal of Abnormal Psychology*, 81: 451–455.

16. Zhong, C-B., Dijksterhuis, A., and Galinsky, A. (2008). The merits of unconscious thought in creativity. *Psychological Science*, 19: 912–918.

17. Rasch, B., and Born, J. (2008). Reactivation and consolidation of memory during sleep. *Current Directions in Psychological Science*, 17: 188–192.

18. Wagner, U., Gais, S., Haider, H., Verleger, R., and Born, J. (2004). Sleep inspires insight. *Nature*, 427: 352–355.

19. Gelbard-Savig, G., Mukamel, R., Malach, R., Harel, M., and Fried, I. (2008). Internally generated reactivation of single neurons in human hippocampus during free recall. *Science*, 322: 96–101. [This is the first study showing reactivation of the same neurons active when a memory was formed in waking when it is recalled sometime later in human patients.]

Chapter 10. The Role of Dreams in the Twenty-four Hour Mind: Regulating Emotion and Updating the Self

1. Jouvet, M. (1999). *The paradox of sleep: the story of dreaming*. Cambridge: Massachusetts Institute of Technology. [Jouvet lays out the basis for his hypothesis that "genetic programming of the brain occurs during paradoxical (REM) sleep. Periodic dreaming would permit the repeated programming of unconscious reactions that are the basis of personality and individual differences in behavior in subjects exposed to the same environments" [pp. 140–141].

2. Damasio, A. (2005). *Descartes' error: emotion, reason and the human brain* (preface ix–xiv). New York: Penguin Books.

3. Payne, J., Stickgold, R., Swanberg, K., and Kensinger, E. (2008). Sleep preferentially enhances memory for emotional components of scenes. *Psychological Science*, 19: 781–788.

4. Pace-Schott, E., Miland, M., Orr, S., Rauch, S., Stickgold, R., and Pitman, R. (2009). Sleep promotes generalization of extinction of conditioned fear. *Sleep*, 32: 19–26.

5. Snyder, F. (1970). The phenomenology of dreaming. In: L. Madow and L. Snow (Eds.), *The psychodynamic implications of the physiological studies on dreams* (pp. 124–151). Springfield IL: Charles Thomas.

6. Cartwright, R., and Lamberg, L. (2000). *Crisis dreaming: using your dreams to solve your problems* (pp. 42–51). Lincoln, NE: ASJA Press. [This is the section on the method of determining the dream dimensions.]

7. Freud, S. (1955). *The interpretation of dreams* (Chapter 7, The psychology of the dream processes, pp. 509-609). New York: Basic Books. [The heart of Freud's theory of dreams is found in Sections D: Arousal by dreams, the function of dreams, anxiety dreams (pp. 573–578) and Section E: The primary and secondary processes-repression (pp. 588–609).]

8. Foulkes, D. (1982). *Children's dreams: longitudinal studies.* New York: John Wiley & Sons.

9. Kagan, J. (2006). *An argument for mind* (p. 126). Princeton, NJ: Yale University Press. [Kagan's studies of the development of temperament in infants through adolescence are summarized in this autobiographical book of his career as a major scientist with a strong point of view about the necessity to observe directly and throw out preconceptions.]

10. Rogers, C. (1951). *Client-centered therapy: its current practice, implications and theory* (Chapter 11: A theory of personality and behavior, pp. 481–533). Boston: Houghton Mifflin Co. [In chapter 11, Rogers develops 19 propositions that form the basis of his theory of the development of normal and abnormal self structures and how they can change based on his clinical experience and research testing of his hypotheses.]

11. Beck, A. (1979). *Cognitive therapy and the emotional disorders.* New York: Penguin Books. [Beck compares and contrasts his cognitive therapy to psychoanalysis. Both attempt to produce structural change by modifying the cognitive organization that produces unrealistic thinking. Cognitive therapy differs in dispensing with abstractions such as id, ego and superego, and the unconscious as antagonistic to the conscious. It treats awareness as a continuum rather than a dichotomy of conscious and unconscious experience.]

12. Giuditta, A., Mandile, P., Montagnese, P., Piscobo, S., and Vescia, S. (2003). The role of sleep in memory processing: the sequential hypothesis. In: P. Maquet, C. Smith, and R. Stickgold (Eds.), *Sleep and brain plasticity* (pp. 157–178). New York: Oxford University Press.

13. Foulkes, D. (1971). The dream-like fantasy scale: a rating manual. *Psychophysiology,* 7: 335–336. [This scale was originally developed to distinguish NREM from REM reports.]

14. Hartmann, E. (1991). *Boundaries in the mind: a new psychology of personality.* New York: Basic Books.

Index